PROGRESS IN HEPATOLOGY 93

British Library Cataloguing in Publication Data
A catalogue record for this book is available from the British Library.

ISBN : 2-7420-0036-4

Éditions John Libbey Eurotext
6, rue Blanche, 92120 Montrouge, France.
Tel. : (1) 47.35.85.52

John Libbey and Company Ltd
13, Smiths Yard, Summerley Street,
London SW18 4HR, England.
Tel. : (1) 947.27.77

John Libbey CIC
Via L. Spallanzani, 11
00161, Rome, Italy.
Tel. : (06) 862.289

PROGRESS IN HEPATOLOGY 93

J.P. MIGUET
D. DHUMEAUX

European Association
for the Study of the Liver
Paris 1993

President : J. P. Benhamou

John Libbey
EUROTEXT

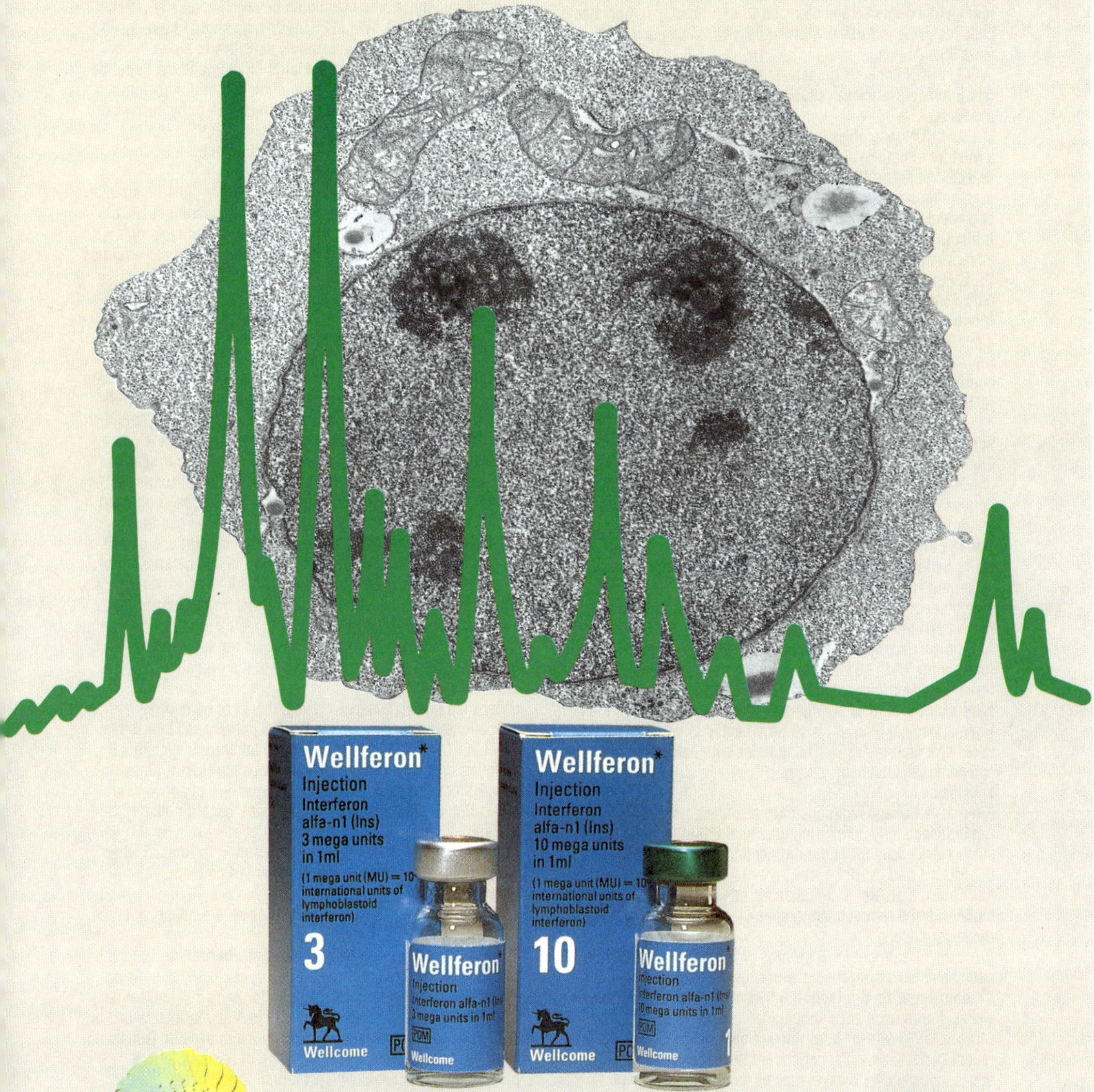
Wellferon*
Injection
Interferon
alfa-n1 (lns)
3 mega units
in 1ml
(1 mega unit (MU) = 10
international units of
lymphoblastoid
interferon)
3
Wellcome
Wellferon
Injection
Interferon alfa-n1
3 mega units in 1ml
POM
Wellcome
Wellferon*
Injection
Interferon
alfa-n1 (lns)
10 mega units
in 1ml
(1 mega unit (MU) = 10
international units of
lymphoblastoid
interferon)
10
Wellcome
Wellferon
Injection
Interferon alfa-n1
10 mega units in 1ml
POM
Wellcome

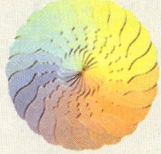

WELLFERON*

Interferon alpha-n1 (Ins)

Presentation Each vial contains either 3 Mega Units or 10 Mega Units of purified WELLCOME human lymphoblastoid interferon, formulated in 1 ml of tris-glycine buffered normal saline in a clear, colourless solution. Albumin Solution Ph. Eur. is included at a concentration of 1.5 mg/ml as a stabiliser.
1 Mega Unit (MU) = 1 x 10^6 International Units (IU) of lymphoblastoid interferon, WHO Reference preparation Ga 23-901-532.

Properties WELLFERON is a highly purified blend of natural human alpha-interferons obtained from human lymphoblastoid cells following induction with Sendai virus. The purity is at least 95%.
WELLFERON contains no detectable DNA (less than 10 picograms of Namalwa cell DNA per millilitre) in the final product.
WELLFERON resembles human leucocyte interferon in that it is a mixture of natural alpha-subtypes; at least 22 have been detected. It also differs from recombinant alpha-interferon preparations made from bacteria or other genetically-engineered cells, which contain only a single subtype.

Indications WELLFERON is indicated for the treatment of patients with hairy cell leukaemia.
WELLFERON is indicated for the treatment of patients with chronic hepatitis B infection.

Mode of Action and Pharmacodynamics The mode of action of alpha-interferon in hairy cell leukaemia is not understood. The rapid rate of clearance of hairy cells from the blood on commencing treatment suggests a direct effect of interferon following cellular binding, particularly since malignant hairy cells are known to bear prolific interferon receptors on their surface membranes.
The mode of action of alpha-interferon in the treatment of chronic hepatitis B infection is poorly understood, but seems to consist of both a direct antiviral effect and immune-modulatory actions.

Dosage and Administration

Hairy cell leukaemia For remission induction, the dose recommended is 3 MU given daily by intramuscular or subcutaneous injection, the latter being more convenient for patient self-administration.
After initial improvement in peripheral haematological indices (commonly 12 to 16 weeks), the dose may be administered thrice weekly, during which time further improvement in the bone marrow is to be anticipated.
Haematological recovery is to be expected in patients who have failed splenectomy as well as in those with palpable splenomegaly in whom reduction in spleen size is to be anticipated.
Alternative dosage regimens have also been used with effect. A randomised study comparing dosing at 2.0 MU/m^2 body surface area daily for one month and then thrice weekly, and 0.2 MU/m^2 body surface area according to the same schedule, has shown a greater anti-leukaemic effect at one year using the higher dosage regimen, although side-effects were less using the lower dose.
Prolonged treatment for 6 months or more may be required to clear hairy cells from the bone marrow.

Chronic hepatitis B infection A twelve-week course of thrice-weekly intramuscular or subcutaneous injections of 10 to 15 MU (up to 7.5 MU/m^2 body surface area) is generally recommended; an initial period, employing escalating daily doses, usually over 5 days, may be a convenient way of introducing treatment.
Longer periods of treatment for up to 6 months at lower doses of 5 to 10 MU (up to 5 MU/m^2 body surface area) thrice weekly have been employed and may be preferred for patients who do not tolerate higher doses.
Some patients appear to be less troubled by interferon-related side-effects if the dose is administered in the evening.

Use in children Dosages of up to 10 MU/m^2 body surface area have been administered to children with chronic hepatitis B infection; however, efficacy of such therapy has not yet been demonstrated. No information is available on the treatment of hairy cell leukaemia in children.
In the rare event of hairy cell leukaemia occurring in children, proportions of the adult dose based on body surface area may be appropriate.

Use in the elderly Elderly patients may be less tolerant of the side-effects of interferon, particularly those effects which are cumulative. These patients should be seen frequently whilst receiving treatment; WELLFERON dosage should be reduced or even stopped if patients are unduly sensitive to side-effects.

Use in immunosuppressed patients Efficacy against hepatitis B virus infection has not yet been demonstrated in patients whose immune systems are compromised (e.g. by current or recent therapy with immunosuppressive drugs (excluding short-term steroid withdrawal) or due to human immunodeficiency virus (HIV) infection).

Pharmacokinetics There is considerable inter-patient variability in the handling of interferons; furthermore, absolute serum levels may be less meaningful as a measure of interferon's biological activity than the induction of certain cellular enzymes such as 2',5'-oligoadenylate synthetase (2-5A synthetase).
Following intramuscular administration, maximum serum levels are usually reached within 4 to 8 hours after dosing, but may merge into a plateau phase as a result of rate-limited absorption from muscle. The measured serum half-life also varies considerably as a result of this, being in the approximate range of 4 to 12 hours, although the true elimination half-life can be estimated to be about 3 to 4 hours. When WELLFERON is administered at the recommended daily dose for the treatment of hairy cell leukaemia, steady state accumulation results in maximum serum values lying in the approximate range of 30 to 90 IU per ml. The range of dosages suggested for the treatment of chronic hepatitis B infection can be expected to result in maximum serum concentrations of 200 to 300 IU per ml. The main route of excretion and catabolism of alpha-interferons is known to be via the kidney following glomerular filtration. In one study, overall body clearance was found to be 57 ml/min/m^2.

Contra-indications WELLFERON should not be given to patients known to be hypersensitive to the preparation or any of its components.
Other than known hypersensitivity, there are no contra-indications to the use of WELLFERON in hairy cell leukaemia.
WELLFERON should not be used to treat chronic hepatitis B infection in patients who have poor hepatic reserve, since successful elimination of serological markers of active viral replication is often preceded by an acute, hepatitis-like illness.

Precautions and Warnings Extreme caution is advised when using alpha-interferons in the treatment of patients with the following:-

concurrent renal, cardiovascular or severe hepatic disease;
central nervous system disease;
a history of pre-existing mental disturbance.

It is important to monitor the blood count closely in patients during the first 6 weeks of treatment for hairy cell leukaemia, following which the suppressive effects of alpha-interferons on the bone marrow will be overtaken by the improving leukaemic state, leading towards a normalisation of haematological parameters. In patients with profound or potentially life-threatening neutropenia or thrombocytopenia at the outset, it may be preferable to initiate treatment using a lower dose of WELLFERON, particularly for out-patients who are remote from immediate medical care.
During WELLFERON treatment of chronic hepatitis B infection, it is important to monitor blood count and liver function

throughout treatment.
Care should be exercised in treating patients with asthma, as exacerbation of the disease has been reported on isolated occasions following alpha-interferon administration.
As alpha-interferons may affect central nervous system functions, patients should be warned not to drive a vehicle or operate machinery until their tolerance of treatment has been assessed.
Carcinogenicity No studies have been conducted in animals to determine whether WELLFERON has carcinogenic potential.
Mutagenicity WELLFERON was not mutagenic in the Ames test.
Teratogenicity Offspring from pregnant rhesus monkeys given daily WELLFERON dosages of up to 2.5 MU/kg (from day 21 through to day 50 in one group and from day 51 through to day 130 in the second group) did not reveal teratogenic or other adverse effects, although there was an increased incidence of abortion and stillbirth in those animals who received the highest dose (2.5 MU/kg daily).
Effects on fertility No studies have been performed in animals to determine whether WELLFERON may affect fertility.
Use in pregnancy and lactation No information is available on the use of WELLFERON in human pregnancy. In view of the profound effects of the drug on human metabolism and physiology however, WELLFERON should be considered as a drug which might result in damage to the foetus, and patients should therefore be advised accordingly. The expected clinical benefit of treatment to the mother must be balanced against any possible risk to the developing foetus. Adequate contraceptive precautions should be advised if either partner is receiving WELLFERON.
In view of the long clinical course of chronic hepatitis B infection and the availability of hepatitis B immunisation for the neonate, use of WELLFERON to treat chronic hepatitis B infection during pregnancy is not recommended.
There is no information on the effects of WELLFERON on human lactation.
Adverse Reactions WELLFERON, in common with other alpha-interferons, is a highly active mediator of biological events and its use may be associated with severe side-effects, particularly when larger doses are administered.
The most frequently reported side-effects of WELLFERON and other alpha-interferon preparations consist of fever, chills, occasionally rigors, headache, malaise and myalgia, all reminiscent of an attack of influenza. These acute side-effects can usually be reduced or eliminated by concurrent administration of paracetamol and tend to diminish with continuing therapy. In contrast however, continuing therapy can lead to lethargy, weakness and fatigue accompanied by anorexia and weight loss.
Alpha-interferons have a suppressive effect on the bone marrow leading to a fall in the white blood count (particularly the granulocytes), the platelet count and, less commonly, the haemoglobin concentration. Additionally, abnormalities in the blood clotting mechanism have occurred. These effects can lead to an increased risk of infection and haemorrhage.
Marked effects on the central nervous system may occur; these include abnormal electroencephalograms with excess slow wave activity, severe depression, confusion, apathy and coma. Occasionally seizures occur, which, in children, may be precipitated by fever. A few reports of movement disorders (including extrapyramidal and cerebellar dysfunction) have been reported in cancer patients receiving WELLFERON.
The administration of alpha-interferons may give rise to hypotension, hypertension, or arrhythmias in certain individuals. Severe cardiovascular events reported in patients receiving alpha-interferons include myocardial infarction, cerebrovascular accident and peripheral ischaemia.
Nausea, vomiting and diarrhoea occur sporadically.
Alpha-interferons can lead to an elevation in liver-related enzymes; this is usually transient but occasionally is marked and persistent. Hepatic necrosis has been reported on very rare occasions.
Rare occurrences of renal failure and/or nephrotic syndrome have been seen in patients treated with WELLFERON. These patients had all been suffering from myelomatosis and had varying degrees of prior renal dysfunction.
Hypocalcaemia and hyperkalaemia have occurred after repeated very high doses (100 – 200 MU) by intravenous infusion.
Reactions at injection sites have been reported in some patients.
Alopecia occurs occasionally as a late side-effect.
Other events which have been reported in patients receiving alpha-interferons include arthralgia, Raynaud's phenomenon, urticaria, erythema nodosum, skin rashes, immune thrombocytopenia, haemolytic anaemia, hypothyroidism, mucositis and isolated peripheral nerve defects, and disturbances of antidiuretic hormone levels.
Drug Interactions Alpha-interferons may alter the activity of certain enzymes. In particular, they reduce the activity of P-450 cytochromes. The metabolism of cimetidine, phenytoin, warfarin, theophylline, diazepam and propranolol by these enzyme systems may therefore be impaired in patients receiving alpha-interferons. Several cytotoxic drugs are also metabolised by these enzymes.
In the treatment of chronic hepatitis B infection, the occurrence of an acute, hepatitis-like illness (see CONTRA-INDICATIONS) presents the theoretical risk of additive interaction with hepatotoxic drugs and of further impairment of hepatic drug metabolism.
Concurrent administration of interferon with drugs which act on the central nervous system has occasionally resulted in unexpectedly severe changes in mental state.
Concurrent administration of immunosuppressive drugs (including corticosteroids), which may enhance viral replication, should be avoided during treatment of chronic hepatitis B infection with WELLFERON.
Overdosage
Symptoms and signs There are no reports of overdosage, but repeated large doses of alpha-interferons are associated with profound lethargy, fatigue, prostration and coma.
Treatment Such patients should be hospitalised for observation and appropriate supportive treatment given.
Pharmaceutical Precautions and Recommendations
Storage precautions Keep at temperatures between 2° and 8°C. Protect from light.
WELLFERON contains no preservative, therefore any partly-used vials should be discarded immediately after withdrawal of the required dose.
Further Information Neutralising antibodies occur infrequently in patients receiving WELLFERON which therefore appears to have low immunogenicity. An overall antibody incidence of 1.8% was found in follow-up sera from more than 900 patients who had received WELLFERON for benign and malignant diseases. In the case of hairy cell leukaemia, no neutralising activity was present in follow-up sera received from over 70 patients despite high, cumulative WELLFERON doses. Following treatment of chronic hepatitis B infection, two of 97 patients (2.1%) developed neutralising antibodies.
The above is the reference Wellcome group datasheet for Wellferon. However, locally, datasheet text will vary in accordance with the regulatory authority requirements/ product licences. Therefore, please consult your local datasheet for detailed prescribing information.

***Trade Mark**
GACT BQGT 91-16

Wellcome

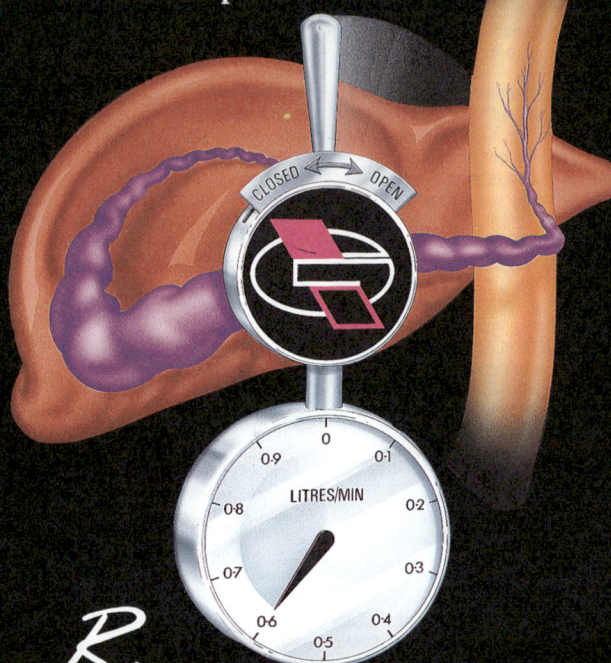

GenHevac B Pasteur

Premier vaccin de 3ème génération

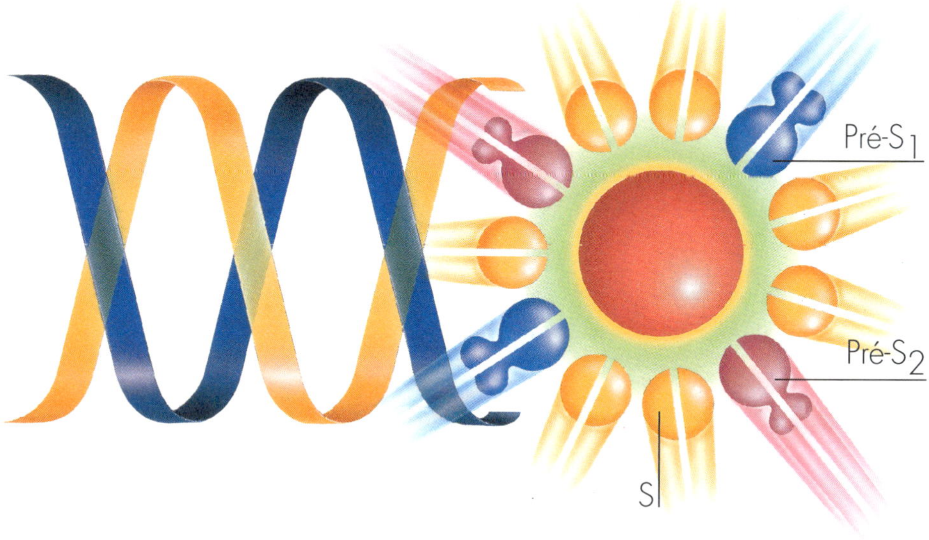

Une protection efficace, précoce et durable contre l'hépatite B.

GENHEVAC B PASTEUR - Vaccin inactivé, purifié, contre l'hépatite B - Description: GenHevac B Pasteur est un vaccin contre l'hépatite B, préparé à partir d'une fraction antigénique on infectante du virus de l'hépatite B (l'antigènique HBs contenant les protéines S et pré-S) produite sur lignée cellulaire CHO. Ce vaccin est obtenu par recombinaison génétique. Les ellules CHO synthétisent et secrétent l'HBsAg sous forme de particules identiques à l'antigène naturel, dont les protéines sont glycosylées et portent les déterminants antigéniques rotecteurs S et pré-S. La préparation est purifiée et inactivée. **Présentation:** Boîte de 1 seringue unidose à usage unique en verre, contenant 0,5 ml de vaccin. **Composition:** Suspension nactivée d'antigène HBs produit sur lignée cellulaire CHO, purifié et contenant : Protéines S et pré-S : 1 dose de vaccin * Hydroxyde d'aluminium (exprimé en aluminium) 1,25 mg naxi) Formaldéhyde 0,10 mg (maxi) Excipient q.s.p. 0,5 ml.*1 dose de vaccin contient 20 µg d'HBsAg. **Propriétés Pharmacologiques:** L'immunité est conférée dans un délai de 1 nois après la 3ème injection. **Indications:** GenHevac B Pasteur a pour indication l'immunisation active contre le virus de l'hépatite B. La vaccination contre l'hépatite B protège ndirectement contre l'infection par le virus delta, virus défectif ne pouvant se répliquer que chez les sujets déjà infectés par le virus HBV. GenHevac B Pasteur ne protège pas contre les épatites infectieuses causées par d'autres agents pathogènes que les virus des hépatites B et delta. Les sujets exposés au risque d'infection par le virus de l'hépatite B comprennent : **ersonnel de santé:** médecins, chirurgiens, infirmières, sages-femmes, biologistes, dentistes, étudiants, personnel d'entretien en milieu hospitalier. **Patients:** hémodialysés, malades olytransfusés. **Sujets vivants en cercle clos:** en particulier prisonniers, handicapés mentaux. **Entourage familial des porteurs de virus:** en particulier nouveau-nés et enfants de mères orteuses du virus. **Sujets séjournants dans les zones de haute endémie:** coopérants, militaires, voyageurs internationaux. **Toxicomanes par voie IV -Sujets à risque en raison de leurs ratiques sexuelles:** homosexuels, prostituées, sujets à partenaires multiples. **Contre-Indications:** Néant. **Précautions d'emploi:** L'expérience acquise avec les vaccins hépatite B dérivés u plasma a montré que les particules d'HBsAg peuvent être administrées sans risque chez la femme enceinte et la femme en période de lactation. Néanmoins, la vaccination avec le GenHevac B Pasteur ne doit être envisagée chez ces sujets que lors d'un risque important d'infection par le virus de l'hépatite B. **Interactions médicamenteuses et autres interactions:** expérience acquise avec les vaccins hépatite B dérivés plasmatiques a montré que : L'administration simultanée du vaccin et d'immunoglobulines spécifiques contre l'hépatite B à ifférents sites d'injection n'entrave pas la réponse immunitaire vis-à-vis du vaccin. L'administration simultanée avec d'autres vaccins (BCG, diphtérie, coqueluche, poliomyélite, tétanos, ougeole, fièvre jaune) n'entrave pas la réponse immunitaire vis à-vis des ces vaccins. L'immunogénicité est diminuée chez les sujets traités par les immunosuppresseurs. **Effets ndésirables:** Aucun effet secondaire grave, locale ou générale et aucune réaction sévère d'hypersensibilité n'ont été rapportés au cours des études cliniques. Les réactions secondaires nodérées suivantes ont été rapportées : Réactions locales : douleurs et induration au point d'injection. Réactions générales : rarement fièvre, myalgie. **Posologie:** Après agitation igoureuse, le vaccin doit être injecté par voie intramusculaire dans le muscle deltoïde chez l'adulte et chez l'enfant à partir de 2 ans ou dans la région quadricipitale haute chez le ouveau-né et l'enfant jusqu'à 2 ans. Le schéma d'immunisation consiste en 3 injections de 0,5 ml, administrées à un mois d'intervalle, suivies d'une injection de rappel 1 an après la re injection, puis d'une injection de rappel tous les 5 ans. Chez les nouveau-nés de mères porteuses d'antigène HBs et/ou d'antigène HBe, il est actuellement recommandé 'administrer simultanément, en deux sites d'injection différents, le vaccin et les immunoglobulines spécifiques anti-hépatite B pour assurer ne protection immédiate. **Conditions de conservation:** Entre +2° C et +8° C. Ne pas congeler. la congélation détruit l'immunogénicité du vaccin.

PASTEUR MÉRIEUX
Sérums & Vaccins

58, AVENUE LECLERC - BP 7056 - 69348 LYON CEDEX 07 - FRANCE

Contents

List of contributors

Alberti A., Clinica Medica II°, University of Padova, Via Giustiniani, 2, 35126 Padova, Italy.

Bailly F., Service d'Hépato-Gastroentérologie, Hôpital de l'Hôtel-Dieu, 69288 Lyon Cedex 2, France.

Berby F., Unité de Recherche sur les Hépatites et les Rétrovirus Humains (INSERM U-271), 151, Cours Albert-Thomas, 69424 Lyon Cedex 3, France.

Berthillon P., Unité de Recherche sur les Hépatites et les Rétrovirus Humains (INSERM U-271), 151, Cours Albert-Thomas, 69424 Lyon Cedex 3, France.

Bismuth H., Hepatobiliary Surgery and Liver Transplant Research Unit, South Paris University, Faculty of Medicine, Hôpital Paul Brousse, 94804 Villejuif, France.

Bonino F., Liver Disease and Laboratory Units of the Department of Gastroenterology, Molinette Hospital, Corso Bramante, 88, 10126 Torino, Italy.

Boudjema K., Centre de Chirurgie Viscérale et de Transplantation, Hôpital de Hautepierre, 67098 Strasbourg Cedex, France.

Brunetto M.R., Liver Disease and Laboratory Units of the Department of Gastroenterology, Molinette Hospital, Corso Bramante, 88, 10126 Torino, Italy.

Camps J., Liver Unit, Hospital Vall d'Hebron, 08035 Barcelona, Spain.

Chiche L., Hepatobiliary Surgery and Liver Transplant Research Unit, South Paris University, Faculty of Medicine, Hôpital Paul Brousse, 94804 Villejuif, France.

Cinqualbre J., Centre de Chirurgie Viscérale et de Transplantation, Hôpital de Hautepierre, 67098 Strasbourg Cedex, France.

Colombo M., Institute of Internal Medicine, University of Milan, Via Pace, 9, 20122 Milano, Italy.

Córdoba J., Liver Unit, Hospital Vall d'Hebron, 08035 Barcelona, Spain.

Dhumeaux D., Service d'Hépatologie et de Gastroentérologie, Hôpital Henri Mondor, 94010 Créteil, France.

Esteban J.I., Liver Unit, Hospital Vall d'Hebron, 08035 Barcelona, Spain.

Habersetzer F., Service d'Hépato-Gastroentérologie, Hôpital de l'Hôtel-Dieu, 69288 Lyon Cedex 2, France.

Hoofnagle J.H., Division of Digestive Diseases and Nutrition, National Institute of Diabetes and Digestive and Kidney Diseases, National Institutes of Health, Bethesda, MD 28092, USA.

Jaeck D., Centre de Chirurgie Viscérale et de Transplantation, Hôpital de Hautepierre, 67098 Strasbourg Cedex, France.

Manns M.P., Department of Gastroenterology and Hepatology, Zentrum Innere Medizin und Dermatologie, Konstanty Gutschow Strasse, 8, D-3000 Hannover 61, Germany.

Mason L.,Gastroenterology Section, Veterans Affairs Medical Center and Washington University School of Medicine, 915 North Grand Boulevard, Saint Louis, MO 63106, USA.

Miguet J.P., Service d'Hépatologie et de Soins Intensifs Digestifs, CHU Jean Minjoz, 25030 Besançon Cedex, France.

Ottobrelli A., Division of Gastroenterology, Molinette Hospital, 10126 Torino, Italy.

Perrillo R.P., Gastroenterology Section, Veterans Affairs Medical Center and Washington University School of Medicine, 915 North Grand Boulevard, Saint Louis, MO 63106, USA.

Pessayre D., Unité de Recherches de Physiopathologie Hépatique (INSERM U-24), Hôpital Beaujon, 92118 Clichy, France.

Pichoud C., Unité de Recherche sur les Hépatites et les Rétrovirus humains (INSERM U-271), 151, Cours Albert-Thomas, 69424, Lyon Cedex 3, France.

Piva A., Institute of Internal Medicine, University of Milan, Via Pace, 9, 20122 Milano, Italy.

Rizzetto M., Institute of Internal Medicine, University of Turin, Cso A.M. Dogliotti, 14, 10126 Turin, Italy.

Shouval D., The Liver Unit, Division of Medicine, Hadassah University Hospital, P.O.B. 12000, 91120 Jerusalem, Israel.

Smedile A., Division of Gastroenterology, Molinette Hospital, 10126 Torino, Italy.

Thomas H., Department of Medicine, St Mary's Hospital Medical School, Norfolk Place, London W2 1PG, England.

Thursz M., Department of Medicine, St Mary's Hospital Medical School, Norfolk Place, London W2 1PG, England.

Trépo C., Service d'Hépato-Gastroentérologie, Hôpital de l'Hôtel-Dieu, 69288 Lyon Cedex 2, France et Unité de Recherche sur les Hépatites et les Rétrovirus humains (INSERM U-271), 151, Cours Albert-Thomas, 69424, Lyon Cedex 3, France.

Vitvitski L., Unité de Recherche sur les Hépatites et les Rétrovirus humains (INSERM U-271), 151, Cours Albert-Thomas, 69424, Lyon Cedex 3, France.

Wolf P., Centre de Chirurgie Viscérale et de Transplantation, Hôpital de Hautepierre, 67098 Strasbourg Cedex, France.

Zafrani E.S., Département de Pathologie, Service d'Anatomie et de Cytologie Pathologiques, Hôpital Henri Mondor, 51, avenue du Maréchal-de-Lattre-de-Tassigny, 94010 Créteil Cedex, France.

Foreword

The publication of the proceedings of the International Post-Graduate Course and the symposia programed in the annual meeting of the European Association for the Study of the Liver — to be supplied to all participants — has been initiated two years ago by Professor J. Rodés and Professor V. Arroyo from Barcelona. No wonder that the torch was lighted by this olympic liver team.

The 1993 International Post-Graduate Course has been designed to provide the hepatologist involved in clinical practice with comprehensive and update reviews on rapidly changing fields of hepatology, like B and C virus liver diseases, benign hepatocellular tumors, drug-induced injury, liver transplantation and preventive medicine. The treatment of chronic viral hepatitis has been chosen as the main theme of the 1993 symposium, as significant advances have been achieved in this important area.

Worldwide hepatologists have all kindly accepted to provide the text of their communications, which represent the main part of this publication. We thank them for their prompt submission and the excellence of their contribution.

Professor J.P. Benhamou, as President, organized the Post-Graduate Course and the symposium with his universally known talent. And thus we are happy to dedicate to him this « Progress in Hepatology 93 ».

Jean-Philippe MIGUET
Daniel DHUMEAUX

Progress in Hepatology 93. J.P. Miguet and D. Dhumeaux, eds.
John Libbey Eurotext, Paris © 1993, pp. 1-11

1

Benign tumours of the liver

E. S. ZAFRANI

Département de Pathologie, Service d'Anatomie et de Cytologie Pathologiques, Hôpital Henri Mondor, 94010 Créteil Cedex, France.

The normal liver is made of various epithelial and mesenchymal cells, and benign tumours may develop from each of these cells [1, 2]. Benign proliferation of the hepatocytes leads to hepatocellular adenoma (HA) and to focal nodular hyperplasia (FNH), in which there is also biliary structure proliferation. Biliary cystadenoma, biliary papillomatosis and bile duct adenoma result from the neoplastic growth of biliary cells. These epithelial lesions are much rarer than hepatic haemangioma, which develops from endothelial cells and constitutes the most common benign tumour of the liver [3]. Other mesenchymal tumours may arise from smooth muscle cells (leiomyoma), fibrocytes (fibroma), adipocytes (lipoma) or nerves (neurofibroma) and some tumours are composed of various cell types, e.g. angiomyolipoma [1, 2].

The purpose of this review is to focus on the main clinico-pathological and radiological findings in haemangioma and in benign epithelial tumours of the liver. These entities raise several questions concerning their pathogenesis and their differential diagnosis from various malignant tumours or pseudotumoral hepatic lesions. Mesenchymal tumours others than haemangioma will not be further considered because of their extreme rarity and pseudotumoral developmental abnormalities such as biliary, endometrial or epidermoid cysts and pancreatic heterotopia will not be included.

Haemangioma

Haemangioma is the most common benign tumour of the liver and its prevalence in the general population is estimated at 0.7 % to 7 % by the study of large autopsy series [3]. Most haemangiomas are small and asymptomatic, and they are incidentally found at ultrasonography (US), laparotomy or *post-mortem* examination of the abdomen [3]. Haemangiomas smaller than 1.5 cm appear as echogenic masses, which is unusual in primary carcinomas or metastatic tumours of the liver [4]. Nuclear magnetic resonance (MR) imaging is very useful when it demonstrates a homogeneous high signal intensity appearance on T2-weighted images [5]. Repeat US within six months may be recommended in order to confirm the benignity of this lesion. Larger haemangiomas are more difficult to diagnose on sonography since they may be hyperechogenic, hypoechogenic or mixed hyper- and hypoechogenic [4]. This heterogeneity is due to possible thrombosis, fibrosis or calcification [1, 2]. In such cases, dynamic computed tomography (CT) before and after contrast medium injection can show characteristic features including : *a*) diminished attenuation on precontrast scan ; *b*) peripheral contrast enhancement during the dynamic bolus phase of scanning ; *c*) isodence fill-in on delayed scans obtained up to 60 min after contrast medium injection [6]. Other diagnostic methods, such as ^{99m}technetium-labelled red blood cells and MR [5], are helpful when these typical and strict haemangioma criteria are not present on CT, which occurs in approximately 45 % of the cases [6].

Whereas small asymptomatic haemangiomas are observed at any age, with the same prevalence in males and females, large haemangiomas are more often symptomatic in women, especially after multiple pregnancies [3]. In addition, occasional reports of large symptomatic haemangiomas in patients receiving oral contraceptives (OC) or oestrogens have been published [7, 8]. These data suggest that, even though these tumours are probably not induced by steroidal compounds, such agents might have a role in the enlargement of a preexisting haemangioma and in the appearance of symptoms. The complications of large haemangiomas are rare ; haemorrhage may occur in approximately 5 % of the cases, being fatal in 2.5 % of them [3]. Taking into account the possible adverse role of oestrogens, the maintenance of OC might be questioned in a woman in whom a haemangioma is incidentally discovered. Since there is no definitive evidence proving that OC are responsible for severe complications, maintenance of OC can be proposed whith regular follow-up by repeated sonographies.

Benign hepatocellular tumours

Focal nodular hyperplasia

Focal nodular hyperplasia (FNH) is a benign tumour that is discovered incidentally in up to 90 % of the cases during physical examination, abdominal imaging work-up, or at laparotomy [9-11]. This lesion, which has also been referred to as focal cirrhosis or hepatic hamartoma, is now considered a tumour-like malformation rather than a neoplasm [12]. Wanless *et al.* [12] have indeed suggested that FNH was secondary to an arterial malformation leading to a hyperplastic response of the liver parenchyma due to increased blood flow. This vascular theory is supported by the association of FNH with other vascular abnormalities, such as telangiectases, hereditary haemorrhagic telangiectasia, arteriovenous malformations and anomalous venous drainage [13]. The association with hepatic haemangioma could represent an additional argument for this theory. In a study including 27 patients with HA and 26 patients with FNH, we have demonstrated the presence of at least one haemangioma on the basis of US, dynamic CT and pathological findings in 23 % of the patients with FNH and in none of the patients with HA [14]. The haemangiomas associated with FNH varied in size, ranging from 1.5 to 4 cm, and were located close or at distance from the FNH [14]. This association had previously been noted in an autopsy study in which haemangiomas were observed in seven of 34 cases (21 %) of FNH [15]. Such a prevalence is markedly higher than the prevalence of 0.7 % to 7 % in the general population [3].

Focal nodular hyperplasia occurs in both sexes and at all ages [16], but most of the cases have been reported in 20 to 50-year-old adults [16]. In addition, females outnumber males by two or more to one [16]. Although the responsibility of oestroprogestatives in the occurrence of the lesion has not been demonstrated, it is possible that these agents or endogenous oestrogens play a role in its enlargement and complications [16, 17].

In approximately 80 % of the cases [11, 18], FNH is a solitary nodule and its macroscopic appearance is highly characteristic. The mass is usually globular, lobulated and well circumscribed, although unencapsulated. Its color is lighter than the surrounding normal liver. The pathognomonic gross feature is the presence, on cut sections, of a central stellate scar with radiating fibrous septa dividing the lesion into nodules. In the recent series published by Vilgrain *et al.*, a scar was observed in 30 of 38 (79 %)

cases ; it was central and solitary in most cases, whereas multiple or peripherally located scars were rarely noted [18]. The tumour is usually small. Among 130 patients with FNH, 110 (84 %) had a single nodule less than 5 cm in diameter, 16 (13 %) had a tumour between 5 and 10 cm, and only 4 (3 %) had a lesion greater than 10 cm [16].

Microscopic examination shows the central stellate fibrous scar irradiating toward the periphery of the tumour and dividing the hyperplastic nodules into smaller units. Marked proliferation of biliary structures surrounded by inflammatory cells is observed within and at the periphery of the fibrous septa. Vascular changes, such as intimal and medial fibromuscular hyperplasia of large vessels in the fibrous scar, sinusoidal dilatation and, very occasionally, haemorrhagic foci or infarction [19], can be noted and are aggravated by the administration of oestroprogestatives [17]. Intake of such agents might favor clinical recognition of the tumour by facilitating its growth and its heamorrhagic complications [14, 20]. This could well explain the higher prevalence of reported cases in women than in men.

To the best of our knowledge, malignant transformation of FNH has never been reported. However, the gross appearance of FNH may resemble that of the fibrolamellar variant of hepatocellular carcinoma [21] and association of these two tumours in close spatial relationship has been recorded [22].

Despite the use of different imaging modalities, FNH may be difficult to differentiate from other hepatic lesions. Ultrasonography is not specific, with various echo patterns [23, 24]. The value of US is its sensitivity for the detection of the lesion. Recently, it has been shown that color Doppler flow imaging could reveal an arterial signal within the tumour, corresponding to the large vessels located in the fibrous scar ; this signal is however not specific of FNH since it is also observed in other tumours including malignant neoplasms (unpublished data). Angiography is now rarely performed. It reveals a hypo- or hypervascular mass with parenchymal staining and, in the majority of the cases, a vascular supply that arises centrally and radiates peripherally in a spokewheel pattern [23, 24]. On CT, FNH is often slightly hypodense prior to contrast medium injection [23, 24]. It may be isodense but, after contrast medium injection, there is marked enhancement at the arterial phase, the lesion becoming isodense in the portal phase and on late scans [23, 24]. The central scar is visualized in 14 % to 43 % of the cases [23, 24]. Scintigraphy may identify normal or increased ^{99m}technetium sulfur colloid uptake because of the presence of Kupffer cells in the tumour [23]. Hepatobiliary scan with trimethylbromoimino-diacetic acid (TBIDA) might be more helpful by demonstrating a hot spot of radioactivity, always present on late images, at 60 min [25]. On MR, which is more and more commonly used, three criteria are considered typical of FNH : *a*) isointensity on T1-and T2-weighted sequences ; *b*) a central hyperintense scar on T2-weighted images ; *c*) a homogeneous signal intensity [26]. In a series above mentioned [18], these typical features were found in 18 of the 42 (43 %) lesions seen at MR ; the remaining 24 lesions had one or more atypical findings including absence of scar (15 cases), hypointense scar on T2-weighted images (7 cases), pseudocapsule (6 cases), strong hyperintense lesion on T2-weighted images (3 cases), diffuse hyperintensity on T1-weighted images (3 cases) and heterogeneity (1 case). In addition, comparison between MR and pathological findings in 38 of these lesions showed that the presence (27 cases) or the absence (8 cases) of a scar on MR was confirmed by the pathological examination ; in three lesions (8 %), a scar less than 4 mm in diameter was not depicted on MR [18]. This comparison also showed that the atypical MR features were related to the existence of foci of haemorrhage, sinusoidal dilatation or abnormal compression of adjacent hepatic parenchyma with mild fibrosis surrounding the lesion [18]. When the MR findings are atypical, the use of new sequences such as ultrafast dynamic snapshot flash imaging might be useful for the analysis of the tumoral vascularization and thus improve the diagnostic performance [27].

Hepatocellular adenoma

Hepatocellular adenoma is a benign proliferation of the hepatocytes within an otherwise normal liver. Although it has occasionally been described in association with type I glycogen storage disease, diabetes mellitus and iron overload secondary to betathalassemia [1], it is now well established that this uncommon tumour occurs, in most of the cases, in women using OC [1, 16, 28]. The incidence is estimated to be 3 to 4 per year per 100,000 long-term OC users, but only 0.1 per 100,000 in non-users or in women who have used OC for less than two years [28]. Furthermore, the risk of developing HA increases with the duration of OC use and with the oestrogen content of OC [28].

In more than 80 % of the cases, patients with HA are symptomatic [1, 11]. Of these, one half have signs and symptoms related to the existence of a mass ; the other half are symptomatic because of haemorrhage, either intratumoral, subcapsular of intraperitoneal [1, 11]. In only 10 %

to 20 % of the patients, HA is incidentally discovered at physical examination, abdominal imaging or laparotomy [1, 11].

Hepatocellular adenoma is usually a solitary spherical nodule, sometimes pedunculated, with a diameter that may reach 30 cm [1]. On cut sections, the tumour is well demarcated from the surrounding liver, being or not encapsulated. Areas of necrosis and/or haemorrhage leading to fibrosis are frequently found. Large blood vessels often run on the surface of the tumour, which thus appears to be vascularized from its periphery [2, 16].

Microscopic examination shows a proliferation of benign hepatocytes that may have an increased content of glycogen and/or fat. Nuclei are generally small and uniform in size but moderately pleomorphic cells with multiple or dysplastic nuclei may be seen in patients who have taken steroids for many years [2]. Non caseating granulomas of unknown cause have been observed in a few cases [16]. Whereas deep in HA, vessels are generally small and normal in appearance, large vessels are noted at the periphery, with changes consisting of intimal thickening of the arteries and smooth muscle hyperplasia of the vein walls. These vascular lesions are aggravated by the administration of OC [17] and are probably responsible for tumour necrosis and occurrence of the life-threatening complications (e.g. intratumoral, subcapsular or intraperitoneal haemorrhage) of this otherwise benign tumour. After withdrawal of OC, the tumour may either regress or, rarely, enlarge [2]. Rare cases of transformation of HA to hepatocellular carcinoma have been reported [29].

Adenomatosis has been defined by the presence of at least 10 HA in an otherwise normal liver and has been regarded as a distinct entity on the basis of the three following arguments : *a*) it affects men as well as women ; *b*) it is unrelated to OC use ; *c*) increases in serum alkaline phosphatase and gamma-glutamyl-transpeptidase are common in adenomatosis but are unusual in HA [30]. The individualization of this entity is debated by some authors who consider it a variant of nodular regenerative hyperplasia of the liver with large nodules [1, 31, 32].

Abdominal US is not specific for HA characterization, since all echostructural patterns (i.e. hypoechoic, hyperechoic, isoechoic or mixed) are observed [24]. The lesion may be anechoic when haemorrhage is marked [24]. As for FNH, the value of US is its sensitivity for lesion detection. Color Doppler flow imaging never reveals arterial within the tumour and this could help in the differential diagnosis with FNH (unpublished data).

On angiography, HA may be either hypovascular with displacement and drapping of hepatic arteries or hypervascular with tortuous vessels coursing through the lesion [33]. Plain CT scans are essential for the detection of intratumoral haemorrhage, which is noted in 15 % of the cases and strongly suggests the diagnosis of HA in a woman using OC [9, 24]. After contrast medium injection, there is significant enhancement at the arterial phase and a decrease during the portal phase, becoming isodense or even hypodense to normal liver within 1 min [24]. The lesions smaller than 4 cm appear homogeneous whereas, in large tumours, hypodense areas corresponding to bands of necrosis with possible fibrous transformation, are frequently observed [24]. Scintigraphy usually identifies a defect on ^{99m}technetium sulfur colloid scans, which has been attributed to a reduced number of Kupffer cells in HA [23]. On MR, tissue characteristics widely vary and HA can be indistinguishable from malignant tumours [33]. When haemorrhagic areas or lipid accumulation in tumour cells are present, hyperintensity is observed on T1-weighted sequences. These sequences rarely show a low intensity pseudocapsule. The hyperintense area on T2-weighted images, which can be observed in FNH, has not been described in HA [33]. This variety of MR findings explains that a specific radiological diagnosis is not possible in HA.

Management of benign hepatocellular tumours

The clinical, radiological, pathological and evolutive differences between FNH and HA must be emphasized since they could have a direct implication on management. Whereas discontinuation of OC, if prescribed, is recommended in these two tumours, their surgical treatment remains controversial and the indication of resection mainly depends on the type of the neoplasm. Indeed, resection is advocated in HA because of the possibility of severe and even fatal complications, such as bleeding, tumour necrosis or transformation into hepatocellular carcinoma. By contrast, FNH might be treated conservatively since it is most often asymptomatic, complications are very rare and no malignant transformation has been recorded. It is therefore of importance to try to get the diagnosis before considering surgery. In a recent study comparing the preoperative and final pathological diagnoses in 51 patients with presumed benign tumours of the liver that have been resected, Belghiti *et al.* [34] showed that : *a*) the affirmation of a preoperative diagnosis of FNH, essentially based on imaging methods, was always confirmed (18 cases) by the pathological examination ; *b*) among the 11 tumours preoperatively diagnosed as HA, 9 were indeed HA and 2 were hepatocellular carcinomas ; *c*) the 22 undetermined lesions corresponded to 18 FNH, 3 HA and 1 hepatocellular carcinoma. These results suggest that, when a diagnosis of FNH is not firmly established preoperatively, laparotomy is mandatory. Frozen sections of a peroperative biopsy can be performed, especially if the tumour is difficult to resect : a diagnosis of HA would incite to remove the lesion, whereas a diagnosis of FNH could lead to temporization.

Benign biliary cell tumours

Biliary cystadenoma

Biliary cystadenoma of the liver is rare and strongly resembles mucinous cystadenoma of the pancreas. Approximately 100 cases have been reported in the literature, and over 85 % of the patients are females more than 30 year-old [1]. This tumour grows progessively and slowly, and clinical findings (i.e. pain, abdominal enlargement, jaundice, nausea or vomiting) depend on the size (2.5 to 25 cm in diameter) and location [1, 35]. CA 19-9 levels may be elevated in the serum and this marker is immunohistochemically detected in biliary tumoral cells [36].

The main pathological feature of biliary cystadenoma is its multilocularity. The locules have various sizes, usually contain a mucinous or gelatinous fluid, and their lining is smooth and thin [35-37]. The cystadenoma is globular in shape and has a smooth external surface. Under light microscopy, the locules are lined by a single layer of normal mucin-producing epithelial cells resting on a layer of highly cellular mesenchymal tissue containing numerous myofibroblasts [38]. Small polypoid or papillary projections may occasionally be observed in the lumen of the locules. The septa between the cavities can be ulcerated and often contain pigment or foamy macrophages, cholesterol clefts, calcifications and various amounts of polymorphous inflammatory cells. Careful examination of the entire tumour is necessary, since foci of adenocarcinoma may arise in an otherwise benign-appearing mucinous cystadenoma [35, 37].

A serous microcystic variety of cystadenoma has been described [2], as in the pancreas. It is made of multiple small cysts lined by a layer of cuboidal epithelial cells that are rich in glycogen and rest on a coat of collagenous tissue. Papillary projections and cellular mesenschymal stroma are not observed in this type of cystadenoma [2].

Biliary papillomatosis

This very rare disorder consists of multicentric intra- and extrahepatic biliary tract adenomatous polypoid tumours with possible transformation into invasive adenocarcinoma [1, 2]. The disease is two times more frequent in men than in women. Patients present with jaundice and die within a few years because of cholangitis, liver failure or carcinomatous transformation. When the disease is limited to one lobe of the liver, radical surgery is possible [1].

Bile duct adenoma

Bile duct adenoma, also termed benign cholangioma or cholangioadenoma, is a rare benign lesion of the liver consisting of the proliferation of non-cystic biliary structures within a dense fibrous stroma [39]. No relationship between this tumour and cholangiocarcinoma has been shown. The small size, the absence of symptoms and its indolent behaviour explain that it is usually discovered during surgery or at autopsy [39]. Its only clinical significance lies in the possible confusion with a well-differentiated adenocarcinoma or with the Von Meyenburg complex, which is a developmental anomaly of small intrahepatic bile ducts [39]. It has recently been reported that some bile duct adenomas contain clusters of endocrine cells that morphologically resemble small metastatic carcinoid tumours and thus may constitute a diagnostic pitfall [40]. In the Allaire *et al.'s* series of 152 cases, the nodules were usually pale, subcapsular, unencapsulated and solitary [39]. Their size ranged from 1 to 20 mm in diameter, with 90 % of the nodules being less than 10 mm. Follow-up of 38 of the surgically treated patients confirmed the benign behaviour of this lesion [39]. The main practical problem raised by this tumour is for the pathologist since its possible discovery during surgery for carcinoma of another abdominal organ leads the surgeon to perform a biopsy for frozen-section diagnosis. The pathologist who is unaware of this rare entity may be puzzled and tempted to call the lesion metastatic carcinoma.

References

1. Goodman ZD. Benign tumors of the liver. In : Okuda K, Ishak KG, eds. Neoplasms of the liver. Tokyo : Springer-Verlag, 1987 : 105-25.
2. Ishak KG. Benign tumors and pseudotumors of the liver. Appl Pathol 1988 ; 6 : 82-104.
3. Zafrani ES. Update on vascular tumours of the liver. J Hepatol 1989 ; 8 : 125-30.
4. Itai Y, Ohtomo K, Araki T, Furui S, Iio M, Atomi Y. Computed tomography and sonography of cavernous hemangioma of the liver. Am J Roentgenol 1983 ; 141 : 315-20.

5. Birnbaum BA, Weinreb JC, Megibow AJ, *et al.* Definitive diagnosis of hepatic hemangiomas : MR imaging versus Tc-99m-labeled red blood cell SPECT. Radiology 1990 ; 176 : 95-101.
6. Freeny PC, Marks WM. Hepatic hemangioma : dynamic bolus CT. Am J Roentgenol 1986 ; 147 : 711-9.
7. Kositchek RJ, Cullen RA. Hemangiomatosis of the liver with thrombosis following use of an oral contraceptive. Calif Med 1970 ; 113 : 70-4.
8. Morley JE, Myers JB, Sack FS, Kalk F, Epstein EE, Lannon J. Enlargement of cavernous haemangioma associated with exogenous administration of oestrogens. S Afr Med J 1974 ; 48 : 695-7.
9. Kerlin P, Davis GL, McGill DB, Weiland LH, Adson MA, Sheedy II PF. Hepatic adenoma and focal nodular hyperplasia : clinical, pathologic, and radiologic features. Gastroenterology 1983 ; 84 : 994-1002.
10. Brady MS, Coit DG. Focal nodular hyperplasia of the liver. Surg Gynecol Obstet 1990 ; 171 : 377-81.
11. Shortell CK, Schwartz SI. Hepatic adenoma and focal nodula hyperplasia. Surg Gynecol Obstet 1991 ; 173 : 426-31.
12. Wanless IR, Mawdsley C, Adams R. On the pathogenesis of focal nodular hyperplasia. Hepatology 1985 ; 5 : 1194-200.
13. Wanless IR, Albrecht S, Bilbao J, *et al.* Multiple focal nodular hyperplasia of the liver associated with vascular malformations of various organs and neoplasia of the brain : a new syndrome. Modern Pathol 1989 ; 2 : 456-62.
14. Mathieu D, Zafrani ES, Anglade MC, Dhumeaux D. Association of focal nodular hyperplasia and hepatic hemangioma. Gastroenterology 1989 ; 97 : 154-7.
15. Feldman M. Hemangioma of the liver. Special reference to its association with cysts of the liver and pancreas. Am J Clin Pathol 1958 ; 29 : 160-2.
16. Ishak KG. Hepatic neoplasms associated with contraceptive and anabolic steroids. In : Lingeman CH, ed. Recent results in cancer research, vol. 66. Berlin : Springer-Verlag, 1979 : 73-128.
17 Nime F, Pickren JW, Vana J, Aronoff BL, Baker HW, Murphy GP. The histology of liver tumors in oral contraceptive users observed during a national survey by the American College of Surgeons Commission on Cancer. Cancer 1979 ; 44 : 1481-9.
18. Vilgrain V, Fléjou JF, Arrivé L, *et al.* Focal nodular hyperplasia of the liver : MR imaging and pathologic correlation in 37 patients. Radiology 1992 ; 184 : 699-703.
19. Brunt EM, Flye MW. Infarction in focal nodular hyperplasia of the liver. A case report. Am J Clin Pathol 1991 ; 95 : 503-6.
20. Zafrani ES, Pinaudeau Y, Dhumeaux D. Drug-induced vascular lesions of the liver. Arch Intern Med 1983 ; 143 : 495-502.
21. Vecchio FM, Fabiano A, Ghirlanda G, Manna R, Massi G. Fibrolamellar carcinoma of the liver : the malignant counterpart of focal nodular hyperplasia with oncocytic change. Am J Clin Pathol 1984 ; 81 : 521-6.
22. Saul SH, Titelbaum DS, Gansler TS, *et al* The fibrolamellar variant of hepatocellular carcinoma. Its association with focal nodular hyperplasia. Cancer 1987 ; 60 : 3049-55.
23. Welch TJ, Sheedy PF II, Johnson CM, *et al.* Focal nodular hyperplasia and hepatic adenoma : comparison of angiography, CT, US, and scintigraphy. Radiology 1985 ; 156 : 593-5.
24. Mathieu D, Bruneton JN, Drouillard J, Caron Pointreau C, Vasile N. Hepatic adenomas and focal nodular hyperplasia : dynamic CT study. Radiology 1986 ; 160 : 53-8.
25. Boulahdour H, Cherqui D, Mathieu D, *et al.* Hot spots in TBIDA liver scan : a constant finding in patients with focal nodular hyperplasia. J Hepatol 1992 ; 16 (suppl. 1) : S34 [abstract].
26. Mattison GR, Glazer GM, Quint LE, Francis IR, Bree RL, Ensminger WD. MR imaging of hepatic focal nodular hyperplasia : characterization and distinction from primary malignant hepatic tumors. Am J Roentgenol 1987 ; 148 : 711-5.
27. Mathieu D, Rahmouni A, Anglade MC, *et al.* Focal nodular hyperplasia of the liver : assessment with contrast-enhanced Turbo FLASH MR imaging. Radiology 1991 ; 180 : 25-30.

28. Rooks JB, Ory HW, Ishak KG, *et al.* Epidemiology of hepatocellular adenoma. The role of oral contraceptive use. J Am Med Ass 1979 ; 242 : 644-8.
29. Gyorffy EJ, Bredfeldt JE, Black WC. Transformation of hepatic cell adenoma to hepatocellular carcinoma due to oral contraceptive use. Ann Intern Med 1989 ; 110 : 489-90.
30. Fléjou JF, Barge J, Menu Y, *et al.* Liver adenomatosis. An entity distinct from liver adenoma ? Gastroenterology 1985 ; 89 : 1132-8.
31. Stromeyer FW, Ishak KG. Nodular transformation (nodular « regenerative » hyperplasia) of the liver. A clinicopathologic study of 30 cases. Hum Pathol 1981 ; 12 : 60-71.
32. Dachman AH, Ros PR, Goodman ZD, Olmsted WW, Ishak KG. Nodular regenerative hyperplasia of the liver : clinical and radiologic observations. Am J Roentgenol 1987 ; 148 : 717-22.
33. Mathieu D, Zafrani ES. Benign tumors of the liver. In : Ferrucci JT, Stark DD, eds. Liver imaging. Current trends and new techniques. Boston : Andover Medical Publishers Inc., 1990 : 177-89.
34. Belghiti J, Pateron D, Panis Y, *et al.* Resection of presumed benign liver tumours. Br J Surg 1993 ; 80 : 380-3.
35. Ishak KG, Willis GW, Cummins SD, Bullock AA. Biliary cystadenoma and cystadenocarcinoma. Report of 14 cases and review of the literature. Cancer 1977 ; 38 : 322-38.
36. Thomas JA, Scriven MW, Puntis MCA, Jasani B, Williams GT. Elevated serum CA 19-9 levels in hepatobiliary cystadenoma with mesenchymal stroma. Two case reports with immunohistochemical confirmation. Cancer 1992 ; 70 : 1841-6.
37. Wheeler DFA, Edmondson HA. Cystadenoma with mesenchymal stroma (CMS) in the liver and bile ducts. A clinicopathologic study of 17 cases, 4 with malignant change. Cancer 1985 ; 56 : 1434-45.
38. Gourley WK, Kumar D, Bouton MS, Fish JC, Nealon W. Cystadenoma and cystadenocarcinoma with mesenchymal stroma of the liver. Immunohistochemical analysis. Arch Pathol Lab Med 1992 ; 116 : 1047-50.
39. Allaire GS, Rabin L, Ishak KG, Sesterhenn IA. Bile duct adenoma. A study of 152 cases. Am J Surg Pathol 1988 ; 12 : 708-15.
40. O'Hara BJ, McCue PA, Miettinen M. Bile duct adenomas with endocrine component. Immunohistochemical study and comparison with conventional bile duct adenomas. Am J Surg Pathol 1992 ; 16 : 21-5.

Progress in Hepatology 93. J.P. Miguet and D. Dhumeaux, eds.
John Libbey Eurotext, Paris © 1993, pp. 13-22

2

Treatment of hepatocellular carcinoma

M. COLOMBO, A. PIVA

Institute of Internal Medicine, University of Milan, Italy.

Ninety per cent of patients with hepatocellular carcinoma (HCC) have associated cirrhosis. Prospective studies of these patients demonstrated that HCC is an asymptomatic and slowly growing tumor whose natural history is an extension of the underlying cirrhosis [1]. There are, however, important variations of the natural history of this tumor in different ethnic groups and between patients. Since the widespread adoption of abdominal ultrasound scan (US) for screening risk patients, the number of patients with early stage tumors who are potentially operable has increased from 10 % to 30 % [2]. However, it is unknown whether mortality from HCC has been reduced in parallel. There are no controlled studies demonstrating the efficacy of any of the available treatments. The efficacy of each treatment modality should be outweighted against the survival of 65 untreated patients with Child-Pugh cirrhosis and a single small tumor, which was 25 % at 3 years.

Patient selection

Patient eligibility for treatment depends upon tumor size and number, and on liver status. To assess the size and number of HCC, lipiodol-arteriography and arterial portography are the first-line preoperative investigations. Because of the great variability in tumor growth, the predictive power of tumor size and number is not absolute. However, the survival times of patients with HCC correlate well with the severity of liver impairment [3]. For staging the clinical status of the patients, the Child-Pugh score system is an accurate assay.

In general, surgery is an option for patients with a single, small tumor and well-preserved hepatic function. For the large number of patients who are not eligible for surgery, percutaneous ethanol injection (PEI) or transcatheter arterial chemoembolization (TACE) have been used as palliative treatments. Pitfalls in patients selection are due to both early tumor spreading to the surrounding liver and to the poor sensitivity of the imaging techniques. Extracapsular microscopic invasion by tumor cells is present in a third of the tumors smaller than 2 centimeters in diameter, as compared to two thirds of those with a larger diameter. As a result, 34 % of the patients with HCC less than 2 centimeters, 41 % of those with 2 to 3 centimeters and 61 % of those with 3 to 5 centimeters, have multiple tumors [4]. The lower prevalence of microscopic tumor invasion from HCC nodes of less than 2 centimetres in diameter led some investigators to restrict the term small HCC to tumors of this size only. Thirty-one per cent of tumors smaller than 2 centimetres escaped US scan detection [5]. Small lesions in the right hepatic lobe and tip of the left hepatic lobe immediately below the diaphragm were overlooked by US scan detection because lung air could interfere. The same is true for HCC presenting as an isoechoic mass. Some lesions also escape detection by CT scan due to overlapping of surrounding organs, the blind area of the interstice gap and the isodense pattern of the tumor. Small tumors with poor vascularity can escape detection by arteriography, but some of them are visualized by arterial portography.

Patients with a single small tumor

Hepatic resection is the primary option for many patients who have a single tumor less than 5 centimeters, well preserved hepatic function and age less than 70 years. Liver transplantation is also considered for younger patients with similar disease including those who have liver function more deteriorated.

Hepatic resection

The functional capacity of the remaining liver is one major factor that affects prognosis for patients undergoing hepatic resection. Thus, less extensive resections are proposed : hepatic segmentectomy and subsegmentectomy are the technical procedures of choice. Between 1978 and 1987, 2 236 Japanese patients, representing 21% of all patients who were diagnosed as having HCC, underwent hepatic resection [6]. The post-operative mortality was 3 % to 11 % and the overall 3-year survival rate was 46 %, including patients with different stages of liver deterioration and tumor size. The best results in terms of both short-term and long-term survival were for the 347 patients (15.5 %) with a single tumor less than 2 centimeters in diameter, for whom the 5-year survival rate was 60.5 % (Table I). Less favourable are the long-term survivals of Western patients which largely result from different criteria for patients selection (Table II). In the Japanese and others' experience, tumor number, infiltration of cancer cells into the fibrous capsule, portal vein invasion by the tumor and tumor growth pattern were other important factors that affected prognoses of the operated patients (Table I).

Table I. Liver Cancer Study Group of Japan : survival rates of 2 236 Japanese patients between 1978 and 1987. Tumor factors associated with outcome of surgery.

Tumor factors		Patients surviving after resection (%)			
		1-yr	2-yr	3-yr	5-yr
Tumor size	2 cm	86.9	81.5	74.5	60.5
	2-5 cm	79.3	67.1	57.4	39.3
	5-10 cm	74.3	57.7	48.0	26.8
Tumor number	Single	80.0	67.8	57.2	38.2
	2 tumors	66.8	48.8	39.9	29.9
Tumor capsule	Infiltrated	76.6	61.2	50.3	34.6
	Not infiltrated	81.3	71.0	61.8	40.1
Portal vein invasion	Present	80.4	69.1	59.8	39.0
	Absent	70.4	52.6	42.9	36.8
Growth pattern	Expansive	81.1	69.1	59.7	41.1
	Infiltrative	65.4	54.9	47.8	27.9
Tumor extent	One segment	85.4	78.7	69.3	53.3
	Two segments	70.0	56.0	51.0	40.0

Table II. Survival of Western patients with cirrhosis and HCC treated by hepatic resection.

Author, year	Center	Era	Patient number	Early mortality (%)	Survival
Bismuth, 1986	Villejuif	70-84	35	14	32 % at 3 yr
Franco, 1990	Villejuif Turin	83-88	72	7	51 % at 3 yr
Ringe, 1991	Hannover	74-78	42	10	18 % at 5 yr
Gozzetti, 1992	Multicenter, Italy	75-88	265	9	46 % at 3 yr

Survival of patients undergoing hepatic resection is influenced not only by the tumor's size and invasiveness, but also by the functional status of the liver expressed as the Child-Pugh score. In fact, the 3-year cummulative survival was 50 % for 78 Japanese patients with a single tumor and Child-Pugh status, 35 % for 26 with Child-Pugh B status and 0 for 3 with Child-Pugh C status [7]. For 72 European patients, these figures were 51 % for Child-Pugh A patients and 12 % for Child-Pugh B-C patients [8]. Thus, there is little evidence supporting treatment by resection of all patients with Child-Pugh B cirrhosis, because of the high risk of operative mortality and the relatively short life expectancy. However, there are exceptions : hepatic resection has been safely performed in patients with HCC in the left lobe of the liver or at the periphery of the right lobe. Resection is contraindicated in patients with Child-Pugh C cirrhosis, due to the high operative risk and the short 6-month life expectancy. The survival of the operated patients appeared to be influenced also by one important technical aspect of surgery, i.e. the margin resection. In one study, 71 patients with a free surgical margin less than 1 centimeter from the tumor's edge in the resected specimens had a 27 % 5-year survival rate, as compared to 64 % for the 37 patients with larger free surgical margins [9]. The outcome of surgery is negatively influenced also by increasing patient age. Patients 65 years of age or older are at risk of intraperitoneal sepsis due to the multiple immunological defects associated with cirrhosis and senescence. Thus, the ideal candidate for hepatic resection is someone less than 65-year old, well-nourished, with Child-Pugh A liver status, who has a capsulated tumor smaller than 2 centimeters and no portal vein infiltration. In this ideal setting, hepatic resection has resulted in a 5-year survival of 78 % [9]. In 223 consecutive patients with HCC seen in Milan in the last 5 years, only 8 % fit these selection criteria. In the study by Sasaki *et al* [10], post-operative mortality, long-term survival and resectability rates were better for 48 patients without cirrhosis than for 142 with cirrhosis. The 9-year survival rates were 57 % and 27 %, respectively. There are several open issues concerning both patients selection and treatment. One such question is the predictive value of the peritumoral fibrous capsule. Though very few patients have completely encapsulated tumors and a capsule free of tumor cells, their survival after hepatic resection is significantly longer than that of other patients. Magnetic resonance imaging seems to be the technique of choice to identify the existence of a capsule.

Another controversy is whether or not preoperative TACE, by reducing the tumor burden, does lower the intraoperative risk of spreading of neoplastic cells. Working against the routine use of TACE in these patients is the 4 % risk of mortality associated with the procedure itself and the lack of evidence that TACE does prolong the survival of patients with unresectable HCC. Another open question is whether or not adjuvant chemotherapy, by eradicating occult nest of tumor cells, improves the survival of resected patients [11].

When liver recurrence or a solitary pulmonary metastasis is detected in a subclinical stage, resection is indicated. Reresection results in a 20 % increase of the 5-year survival after radical resection of HCC [12]. In non-resectable patients, TACE and PEI have been used to treat intrahepatic recurrences.

Orthotopic liver transplantation (OLT)

In selected patients with a small HCC, the major advantage of OLT is that it removes both detectable and undetectable tumor nodes together with all the preneoplastic lesions that are present in the cirrhotic liver. Moreover, removal of the diseased liver reduces the risk of morbidity and mortality from portal hypertension, which is high in patients with thrombosis of the portal vein trunk. However, opposing these « pros » for OLT are several important « cons », including shortage of donated organs, stringent criteria of patient selection, early mortality for HBV-infected patients and high risk of early tumor recurrence due to immunosuppression. More recently, the overall patient survival following OLT has improved markedly since the introduction of cyclosporine and accurate criteria of patient selection (Table III). In Hannover, the 3-year survival of patients transplanted for malignant hepatobiliary disease was 15 % in 1975-1983, as compared to 45 % in 1984-1987 [13]. In Pittsburgh, 5-year survivals of 45 % were achieved [14] in patients with single small tumors. However,

Table III. Survival of transplanted patients with HCC.

Author, year	Center	Era	Patient number	Early mortality	Survival (%)		
					1 yr	3 yr	5 yr
O'Grady, 1989	Cambridge/KCH	68-86	19	21	45	35	35
Jenkins, 1989	Boston	83-87	8	15	50	-	-
Yokoyama, 1990	Pittsburgh	80-88	80	-	64	45	45
Wolf, 1989	Berlin	-	18	-	50	18	-
Olthoff, 1990	Los Angeles	84-89	16	25	40	-	-
Ringe, 1991	Hannover	74-88	67	15	38	15	15
Moreno, 1992	Madrid	86-90	12	0	64	-	-

the best long-term survivals were in patients in whom HCC was not the primary indication for OLT but was discovered by chance during examination of the explanted liver. In Pittsburgh, the 5-year survival of 16 such patients who underwent transplantation for chance-discovered HCC was 90 %. Thus, the survival of the transplanted patients is largely influenced by tumor size and number, as is the survival of resected patients with HCC. In 62 patients with non-fibrolamellar HCC studied by Yokoyama in Pittsburgh, the tumors less than 5 centimeters in the largest diameter recurred less frequently than larger tumors (7 % *vs* 62 %, $p<0.05$). The same was true for tumors without gross vascular invasion as compared to those with gross vascular invasion (29 % *vs* 73 %, $p < 0.05$). Investigation of perihepatic lymph nodes is another crucial step of tumor staging : it is carried out preoperatively by CT scan and/or laparoscopy or during laparotomy. In Hannover, the overall 5-year survival in 67 patients who were transplanted between 1974 and 1988 was 15 % but it was 60 % for patients with solitary small HCC and no lymph node metastases [13]. Similar results were obtained in Pittsburgh. Thus, although criteria for patient selection varied from center to center, many agree that the ideal candidate for OLT is a patient less than 60-year old with a tumor smaller than 3 centimeters and with no vascular or perihepatic lymph nodes invasion. The most common cause of early death, i.e. within 3 months after OLT, is graft failure. The most common cause of late death, i.e. 3 months after OLT, is recurrence of the original tumor. There are several open questions about OLT treatment of patients with HCC. One such question is how to reduce the risk of treatment failure, i.e. tumor recurrence. In many instances, tumor recurrence results from faulty pretransplant evaluation of the patients, due to the poor sensitivity of the currently available imaging techniques. Tumor recurrence can also be caused by enhanced tumor growth under immunosuppressive therapy. In a study of 9 patients with recurrent HCC, the tumor doubling time was 26 ± 11 days for those patients on cyclosporine-steroid therapy, as compared to the average 6 months reported in the literature [14]. Another open question is the potential usefulness of adjuvant chemotherapy. One currently employed schedule of treatment is epidoxorubicin given at doses of 20 to 30 mg at weekly intervals for 10 weeks. However, there are no controlled data demonstrating that the risk of tumor recurrence in transplanted patients is lowered by this treatment.

Patients with advanced disease

Many patients with single HCC are rejected for surgery because of either advanced liver replacement by tumor or deteriorated liver status. There are also patients who fit the criteria for surgery but who are rejected because of advanced age, extrahepatic disease, strategic tumor localization or a combination of these factors. For this heterogeneous group of « non-operable » patients, there are several different treatments available.

Percutaneous ethanol injection (PEI)

Treatment of a small HCC by PEI is possible because ethanol causes extensive cellular coagulative necrosis, diffuses selectively into the neoplastic tissue, and is well tolerated. Patients eligible for PEI are those with a single lesion less than 5 centimeters in diameter, no extrahepatic metastases and Child-Pugh A or B liver status. In four controlled studies, up to 73 % of the lesions treated by PEI underwent complete coagulative necrosis and 68 % to 80 % of the patients were alive 3 years after onset of therapy (Table IV) [15-19]. As for surgery, patient survival depended upon three factors : tumor size, tumor number and liver status. The 2-year survival was 100 % for Japanese patients with a tumor smaller than 2 centimeters, as compared to 75 % for the general population of patients. Similarly, all 6 Spanish patients with tumors smaller than 2 centimeters were tumor-free and alive 4 to 21 months following PEI as compared to 28 % of the patients with HCC between 2 and 3 centimeters, and 91 % of those with larger tumors. In a multicenter Italian study of 207 patients [17], the 3-year survival of patients with 2 or 3 tumor nodes was less than that for patients with a solitary tumor (31 % *vs* 63 %). The same was true for patients with Child-Pugh class B/C as compared to patients with Child-Pugh A (42 % and 0 *vs* 76 % respectively). Similar data were obtained in 75 Japanese patients, in whom the 3-year survivals were 72 % for Child-Pugh A, 77 % for Child-Pugh

Table IV. Survival of patients with a single HCC treated by percutaneous ethanol injection.

Author, year	Center	Patient number	Survival (%)		
			1 yr	2 yr	3 yr
Ohto, 1987	Chiba	21	–	86	80
Seki, 1989	Osaka	18	–	75	–
Ebara, 1990	Tokyo	75	93	81	65
Livraghi, 1992	Multicenter North Italy	162	90	80	63
Bruix, 1992	Barcelona	24	80	60	50
Marin, 1992	Padova	57	94	85	60

B and 28 % for Child-Pugh C patients [19]. Data from all these studies are against the use of PEI for patients with Child-Pugh C liver status. Instead, life expectancy of Child-Pugh A patients with small tumors treated by PEI appears to be as good as that for similar patients who are treated by hepatic resection. Since the safety and costs of these two treatments differ appreciably, a randomized clinical trial comparing the efficacy of these two treatment modalities in Child-Pugh A patients appears worthwhile to many.

Transcatheter arterial chemoembolization

Despite the plethora of publications on TACE, almost all the results are based on anedoctal reports or uncontrolled studies. Despite the fact that an objective response is often seen, significant prolongation of median survival has not been demonstrated. Repeated arterial embolization is more effective in causing tumor necrosis than single embolization [20]. The 1, 2 and 3-year survival of 1 061 Japanese patients with unresectable HCC treated by TACE were 51, 20 and 13 % [21]. Similarly disappointing results were obtained in Western patients [22]. One major drawback of TACE is the so-called post-embolization syndrome, i.e. intermittent fever, abdominal pain, nausea and vomiting, and abdominal fullness, which affects almost all patients and sometimes lasts 1 to 2 weeks. In 15 % of these patients, severe symptoms develop as a consequence of gallbladder infarction resulting from cystic artery embolization, or pancreatitis resulting from pancreatic artery embolization. TACE is contraindicated for patients with a venous tumor supply, more advanced liver deterioration, thrombosis of the portal vein trunk or renal failure.

Other palliative treatments

Systemic chemotherapy has been widely used to treat inoperable patients with HCC, with a very low response rate. In the only randomized controlled trial [23], doxorubicin not only failed to prolong patients' survival but also caused fatal complications due to cardiotoxicity in 18 % of them. The possible sex hormone dependence of HCC and the presence of tumor hormone receptors have suggested to several investigators a potential for hormonal manipulation of tumor growth. However, preliminary studies with tamoxifen gave conflicting results. Palliative radiotherapy for pain reduction has been attempted by whole liver irradiation at under 25 Gy over 5 to 6 weeks, which was considered the minimum required to control HCC [24].

Conclusions

Tumor size and number, and liver status are common guidelines for selecting patients for treatment. Hepatic resection and liver transplantation are the best chances of cure for selected patients with a single small tumor. In those patients, 3-year survival is longer than that of historical controls, which is 25 % for Child-Pugh A patients. At this point, a controlled study comparing the cost-efficacy of resection and transplantation is seemed necessary by many. Less satisfactory is the long-term outcome of surgery in patients with tumor spreading to the surrounding liver and perihepatic lymph nodes. Patients with more advanced disease have dismal prognoses. For some of these patients, particularly those with tumors less than 5 centimeters in diameter who are not eligible for surgery, PEI appears to be cost-effective. It is still uncertain whether or not TACE is an actually cost-effective treatment for non-operable patients.

References

1. Okuda K. Hepatocellular carcinoma : recent progress. Hepatology 1992 ; 15 : 848-963.
2. Colombo M, de Franchis R, Del Ninno E, *et al.* Hepatocellular carcinoma in Italian patients with cirrhosis. N Engl J Med 1991 ; 325 : 675-80.
3. Okuda K, Ohtuki T, Obata H, *et al.* Natural history of hepatocellular carcinoma and prognosis in relation to treatment. Cancer 1985 ; 56 : 918-28.
4. Otho M, Kondo F, Ebara M. Pathology, diagnosis and treatment of small liver cancer. In : Tobe T, Kaneda H, Okudaira M, Otho M, Endo Y, Mito M, Okamoto E, Tarikawa K, Koijro M, eds. Primary liver cancer in Japan. Tokyo, Berlin, Heidelberg, New York, London, Paris, Hong-Kong, Barcelona : Springer, 1992.
5. Choi BI, Han JK, Song IS, *et al.* Intraoperative sonography of hepatocellular carcinoma : detection of lesions and validity in surgical resection. Gastrointest Radiol 1991 ; 16 : 329-33.
6. Tobe T, Arii S. Improving survival after resection of hepatocellular carcinoma : characteristics and current status of surgical treatment of primary liver cancer in Japan. In : Tobe T, Kaneda H, Okudaira M, Otho M, Endo Y, Mito M, Okamoto E, Tarikawa K, Koijro M, eds. Primary liver cancer in Japan. Tokyo, Berlin, Heidelberg, New York, London, Paris, Hong-Kong, Barcelona : Springer, 1992.
7. Nagasue N, Yukaya H. Liver resection for hepatocellular carcinoma : results from 150 consecutive patients. Cancer Chemother Pharmacol 1989 ; 23 : S78-82.
8. Franco D, Capussoti L, Smadja C, *et al.* Resection of hepatocellular carcinoma. Results in 72 European patients with cirrhosis. Gastroenterology 1990 ; 98 : 733-8.
9. Yamanaka N, Okamoto E. Conditions favoring long-term survival after hepatectomy for hepatocellular carcinomas. Cancer Chemother Pharmacol 1989 ; 23 : S83-6.
10. Sasaki Y, Imaoka S, Masutani S, *et al.* Influence of coexisting cirrhosis on long-term prognosis after surgery in patients with hepatocellular carcinoma. Surgery 1992 ; 112 : 515-21.
11. Hamada T, Shigemura T, Kodama S, *et al.* Hepatic resection is not enough for hepatocellular carcinoma. A follow-up study of 92 patients. J Am Gastroenterol 1992 ; 14 : 245-50.
12. Tang ZY, Yu Y, Zhon XD, *et al.* Surgery of small hepatocellular carcinoma. Analysis of 144 cases. Cancer 1989 ; 64 : 536-41.
13. Ringe B, Pichlmayr R, Wittekind C, Tush G. Surgical treatment of hepatocellular carci-

noma : experience with liver resection and transplantation in 198 patients. World J Surg 1991 ; 15 : 270-85.
14. Van Thiel DH, Carr BI, Yokoyama I, *et al.* Liver transplantation as a treatment of hepatocellular carcinoma. In : Tobe T, Kaneda H, Okudaira M, Otho M, Endo Y, Mito M, Okamoto E, Tarikawa K, Koijro M, eds. Primary liver cancer in Japan. Tokyo, Berlin, Heidelberg, New York, London, Paris, Hong-Kong, Barcelona. Springer, 1992.
15. Sugiura N, Takara K, Otho M, *et al.* Treatment of small hepatocellular carcinoma by percutaneous injection of ethanol into tumor with real-time ultrasound monitoring. Acta Hepatol Jpn 1983 ; 24 : 920-8.
16. Shiina S, Yasuda H, Muto H, *et al.* Percutaneous ethanol injection in the treatment of liver neoplasms. Am J Roentgenol 1987 ; 149 : 949-52.
17. Livraghi T, Bolondi L, Lanzani S, *et al.* Percutaneous ethanol injection in the treatment of hepatocellular carcinoma in cirrhosis. A study of 207 patients. Cancer 1992 ; 69 : 925-9.
18. Vilana R, Bruix J, Bru C, *et al.* Tumor size determines the efficacy of percutaneous ethanol injection for the treatment of small hepatocellular carcinoma. Hepatology 1992 ; 16 : 353-7.
19. Ebara M, Otho M, Sugiama N, *et al.* Percutaneous ethanol injection for the treatment of small hepatocellular carcinoma. Study of 95 patients. J Gastroenterol Hepatol 1990 ; 5 : 616-26.
20. Lin DY, Liaw YF, Lee TY, *et al.* Hepatic arterial embolization in patients with unresectable hepatocellular carcinoma. A randomized controlled trial. Gastroenterology 1988 ; 94 : 453-6.
21. Yamada R, Kishi K, Terada M, *et al.* Transcatheter arterial chemoembolization for unresectable hepatocellular carcinoma. In : Tobe T, Kaneda H, Okudaira M, Otho M, Endo Y, Mito M, Okamoto E, Tarikawa K, Koijro M, eds. Primary liver cancer in Japan. Tokyo, Berlin, Heidelberg, New York, London, Paris, Hong-Kong, Barcelona : Springer, 1992.
22. Pelletier G, Roche A, Ink O, *et al.* A randomized trial of hepatic arterial chemoembolization in patients with unresectable hepatocellular carcinoma. J Hepatol 1990 ; 11 : 181-4.
23. Lai C, Wu P, Chan G, *et al.* Doxorubicin *versus* no antitumor therapy in inoperable hepatocellular carcinoma. A prospective randomized trial. Cancer 1988 ; 62 : 479-83.
24. Nagata Y, Abe M, Hiraoka M, *et al.* Radiofrequency hyperthermia and radiotherapy for hepatocellular carcinoma. In : Tobe T, Kaneda H, Okudaira M, Otho M, Endo Y, Mito M, Okamoto E, Tarikawa K, Koijro M, eds. Primary liver cancer in Japan. Tokyo, Berlin, Heidelberg, New York, London, Paris, Hong-Kong, Barcelona : Springer, 1992.

Progress in Hepatology 93. J.P. Miguet and D. Dhumeaux, eds.
John Libbey Eurotext, Paris © 1993, pp. 23-39

3

Toxic and immune mechanisms leading to acute and subacute drug-induced liver injury

D. PESSAYRE

Unité de Recherches de Physiopathologie Hépatique (INSERM U-24), Hôpital Beaujon, 92118 Clichy, France.

During the process of evolution, animals were subjected to a biological warfare mounted by the plants that they ingested. By duplication of an ancestral gene, divergence of these 2 genes, and so forth, surviving animals are now endowed with multiple cytochromes P-450 which can metabolize (and thus eliminate) liposoluble xenobiotics (including present day drugs). Cytochrome P-450 transforms some drugs into chemically reactive metabolites. These free radicals or electrophilic metabolites attack hepatic constituents. When this attack is extensive, toxic hepatitis ensues. The susceptibility of some subjects (idiosyncrasy) may be due to acquired (e.g. induction, denutrition) or genetic factors (e.g. deficit in glutathione synthetase). When the formation of reactive metabolites is moderate, severe toxic lesions do not occur. However, the covalent binding of reactive metabolites onto hepatic proteins (« alkylated » proteins) modifies the « self » of the subject. In some subjects, this triggers immunization against either normal epitopes (autoimmune reaction) or epitopes modified by the attachment of a reactive metabolite (modified self). Both genetic defects in protective mechanisms (leading to extensive alkylation) and the HLA phenotype modulate the likelihood of immunization. Several drugs inhibit the mitochondrial β-oxidation of fatty acids ; these are esterified into triglycerides which accumulate as small lipid droplets, leading to microvesicular steatosis. Other drugs decrease the extrusion of triglycerides from the liver and lead to macrovacuolar steatosis. Pseudo-alcoholic liver lesions are seen with cationic amphipilic drugs which enter the mitochondria along the mitochondrial membrane potential, reach high intramitochondrial concentrations, and inhibit both the respiratory chain (leading to decreased ATP and cell necrosis) and β-oxidation (leading to steatosis). Steatosis may lead to lipid peroxidation, releasing both chemoattractants (responsible for polymorphonuclear cell infiltration) and malondialdehyde (possibly cross-linking cytokeratins and forming Mallory bodies).

Although several hundred drugs are hepatotoxic, the mechanisms of drug-induced liver injury have only been studied for a few drugs [1]. The same drug may damage the liver by various mechanisms, leading to diverse lesions in different patients [1]. Despite these difficulties, a global picture is nevertheless emerging of the main mechanism(s) responsible for each type of liver lesion. The present chapter summarizes the mechanisms involved in acute and subacute drug-induced liver injury. A more comprehensive survey has been published [1].

Acute hepatitis

Liver lesions consist of lobular and portal inflammation, with lobular liver cell necrosis (« cytolytic hepatitis »), cholestasis (« cholestatic hepatitis »), or both (« mixed hepatitis ») [2]. One mechanism appears to be particularly frequent, namely the formation of reactive metabolites (Figure 1).

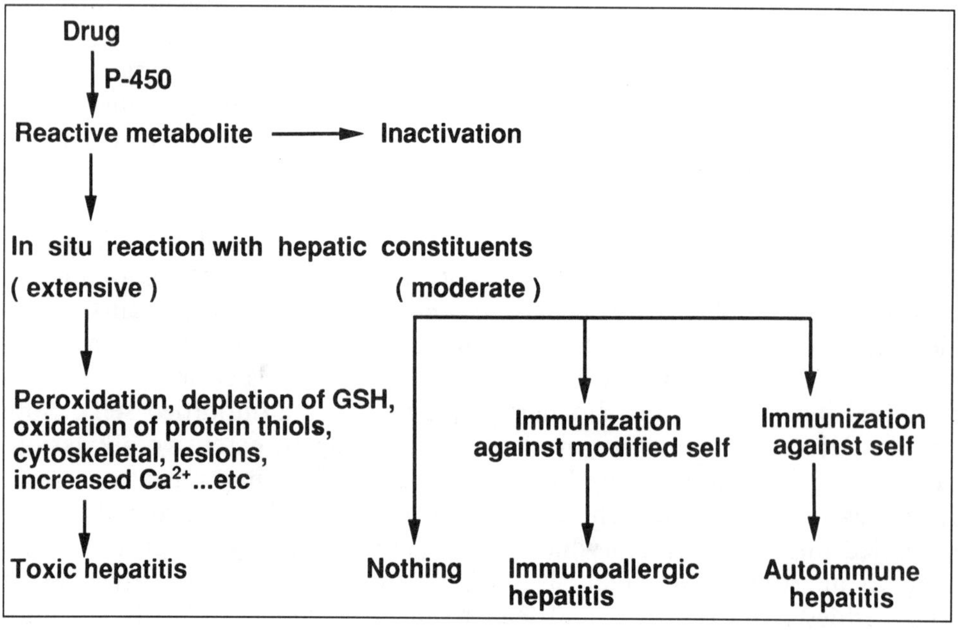

Figure 1. Toxic and immune mechanisms leading to acute drug-induced hepatitis.

Formation and inactivation of reactive metabolites

During the millennia of evolution, animals were subjected to a relentless biological warfare mounted by the plants that they ingested, as these plants progressively developed new liposoluble toxic substances [3]. By duplication of an ancestral gene, divergent evolution of these 2 genes, and so forth, surviving animals are now endowed with multiple cytochromes P-450 which can metabolize (and thus eliminate) environmental liposoluble xenobiotics. Cytochrome P-450 oxidizes these xenobiotics, while conjugating enzymes add a polar, water-soluble group. The hydrosoluble conjugate is then eliminated in urine or bile. Likewise, many drugs are lipophilic and require conversion to water-soluble metabolites to be eliminated.

After reduction by NADPH-cytochrome P-450 reductase, cytochrome P-450 binds molecular oxygen as a sixth ligand of its haem iron. After a second electron is introduced, a reactive iron oxo complex is formed which can oxidize many substrates [4]. While some drugs are transformed into stable metabolites, other drugs form reactive, potentially toxic, metabolites (Figure 1).

Toxicity is fortunately limited by several protective mechanisms [1]. A reactive intermediate which has just been formed inside the hydrophobic pocket of cytochrome P-450 may inactivate cytochrome P-450. This limits the formation and toxicity of the metabolite. Epoxide hydrolases convert many reactive epoxides into inactive dihydrodiols. Most electrophilic metabolites are conjugated with glutathione (GSH) and thereby detoxified. This spontaneous reaction is further catalysed by several cytosolic and microsomal GSH S-transferases.

Other systems limit the toxicity of reactive oxygen species or prevent lipid peroxidation [1]. Thanks to the combined action of these protective mechanisms, only a small fraction of the administered dose will ultimately damage hepatic constituents.

In situ reaction of reactive metabolites

While some slightly reactive metabolites, such as acetaldehyde or acylglucuronides, may leave their site of formation and react elsewhere, most reactive metabolites are so unstable that they mainly react *in situ* in the organ that forms them. The abundance of cytochrome P-450 in the liver, and the *in situ* reaction of reactive metabolites explains the unique role of these metabolites in drug-induced hepatitis. Centrilobular hepatocytes, which contain high levels of cytochrome P-450 and low levels of the protective GSH, are selectively affected [1]. The reaction of reactive metabolites with hepatic constituents may produce hepatitis by either toxic or immune mechanisms (Figure 1).

Toxic hepatitis produced by reactive metabolites

The reaction of the metabolite with hepatic constituents may lead to several molecular lesions (Figure 1). One type, seen with free radicals, is lipid peroxidation [1]. Either the addition of a drug free radical (R°) on a carbon of an unsaturated lipid, or the abstraction by this radical of an hydrogen atom from this lipid, leads to a lipid radical (L°). This radical then quickly adds molecular oxygen to form a peroxyl radical (LOO°). This first peroxyl radical ($Lipid_1$-OOH) may react with another lipid molecule ($Lipid_2$-H) to form a hydroperoxide ($Lipid_1 - OOH$) and a new lipid radical ($Lipid_2$° : $Lipid_1$-OO° + $Lipid_2$-H → $Lipid_1$-OOH + $Lipid_2$°. Lipid peroxidation may thus extend from one lipid to the other, or along the same lipid chain. Although hydroperoxides are relatively stable, they can reform highly reactive radical species, such as alkoxy radicals (LO°), in the presence of ferrous iron. Alkoxyl radicals may split, with the formation of two fragments : an aldehyde and an ethyl or pentyl radical (leading to the exhalation of ethane and pentane). Thus, unsaturated lipids are oxidized and cut into small fragments (alkanes, malondialdehyde, alkenals). The last two compounds are themselves reactive, and covalently bind to proteins.

A second molecular lesion, which occurs mostly with electrophilic metabolites, is the covalent binding of the metabolite to different nucleophilic sites of proteins (e.g. the SH group of a cysteine residue, or the ϵ-NH_2 group of a lysine residue), nucleic acids or both.

A third molecular lesion is the depletion of GSH. Electrophilic metabolites react with the nucleophilic SH group of GSH. This conjugation has an important protective effect, as long as it does not exceed the capacity of the liver to resynthesize GSH. When the formation of the electrophilic metabolite is very high, consumption of GSH leads to GSH depletion. This has three major toxicological consequences : *a)* once GSH is depleted, reactive electrophilic metabolites cannot bind to GSH, and bind massively to hepatic proteins ; *b)* depletion of GSH compromises antioxidant protective mechanisms, and therefore permits the onset of lipid peroxidation ; *c)* depletion and/or oxidation of GSH leads to the oxidation of protein thiols [1].

Oxidation of protein thiols impairs the function of several critical proteins. Actin is the building block of microfilaments, which form a dense network under the plasma membrane surface. By interacting with plasma membrane proteins, microfilaments help to maintain the shape of this membrane. Actin has several reactive SH-groups. During oxidative stress, these groups are oxidized to disulfide bridges which link several molecules of actin, and form large macromolecular aggregates [5]. Disruption of the microfilamentous network permits the formation of plasma membrane blebs. Rupture of a large bleb releases the cell content in the extracellular milieu, and leads to cell death. A second molecular consequence of the oxidation of protein thiols (particularly in the presence of high concentrations of Ca^{2+}) is to damage and permeabilize the inner mitochondrial membrane, causing the collapse of the mitochondrial membrane potential, and depriving the cell of energy [6]. A third consequence of the oxidation of protein thiols is to increase cytosolic calcium [7]. Normally, the intracytoplasmic concentration of ionized calcium is maintained at low levels by plasma membrane calcium translocases which utilize the energy fo ATP to extrude Ca^{2+} from hepatocytes. Oxidation of the protein thiols of calcium translocases damages these carriers [7]. Decreased extrusion of calcium, together with the increased entry of calcium through the damaged plasma membrane, and decreased sequestration of calcium in the endoplasmic reticulum and mitochondria, all produce a marked and sustained increase in cytosolic Ca^{2+} concentration. This in turn activates phospholipase A2, calcium-dependent proteases (which participate in the disruption of cytoskeletal proteins) and nuclear endonucleases (which cut DNA between nucleosomes) [7]. These various changes eventually lead to cell death and cytolytic hepatitis (Figure 1).

Clinical aspects of toxic hepatitis

Toxic drug-induced hepatitis is not associated with hypersensitivity manifestations [2]. It does not occur more quickly after a rechallenge than after the first administration. Toxic drug-induced hepatitis, however, has not the predictability usually expected from a toxic phenomenon. Obviously, a molecule that would produce constant hepatitis at therapeutic doses during clinical trials would not be placed on the market. Instead, drug-induced toxic hepatitis occurs in only a few patients receiving therapeutic doses. Both acquired and genetic factors may explain this apparent idiosyncrasy.

Acquired factors influencing toxic hepatitis

Pregnancy decreases the capacity of the liver to resynthesize GSH, and markedly increases the hepatoxicity of paracetamol in mice [8]. It is unknown whether similar effects occur in humans. Fasting or protein denutrition decreases hepatic GSH content, and dramatically increases the hepatotoxicy of paracetamol in rats [9] and in humans [2].

Microsomal enzyme induction by drugs administered concurrently may increase the formation of the reactive metabolite, and the susceptibility to hepatitis. Thus, rifampicin and other microsomal enzyme inducers apparently increased the hepatotoxicity of isoniazid [10]. Recent introduction of microsomal enzyme inducers may have triggered fulminant hepatitis in three patients receiving iproclozide [11]. Chronic ethanol ingestion increases cytochrome P-450 2E1 which metabolizes ethanol, but also paracetamol. Induction of this isoenzyme potentiates the hepatotoxicity of therapeutic doses of paracetamol in alcohol-abusers [12]. Ethanol consumption also tends to decrease hepatic GSH concentration [13], an effect which may also contribute to increased paracetamol toxicity. Indeed, inducers and fasting had additive effects on the hepatotoxicity of paracetamol in rats [14].

Genetic factors influencing toxic hepatitis

A genetic deficiency in cytochrome P-450 2D6 or in a form of cytochrome P-450 2C which metabolizes mephenytoin is observed in certain subjects [15]. These subjects should be protected against the toxicity of those reactive metabolites which happen to be formed mainly by the deficient cytochrome P-450 isoenzyme. Statistically, however, most reactive metabolites are likely to be formed by other isoenzymes of cytochrome P-450 [16].

Genetic defects in protective mechanisms may increase toxicity. Subjects with a deficiency in GSH synthetase were less able to increase the resynthesis of GSH than normal subjects, and were thus more susceptible to paracetamol toxicity, at least in an artificial *in vitro* system [17].

Relative rarity of toxic drug-induced hepatitis

Preclinical toxicological studies and premarketing clinical trials usually disclose and eliminate most, if not all, molecules with a direct toxic potential. This tends to eliminate drugs that produce toxic liver injury. Current premarketing studies, however, do not eliminate drugs which form reactive metabolites in low amounts, amounts insufficient to directly damage hepatocytes by a toxic mechanism. Such drugs do not produce toxic hepatitis (Figure 1). Covalent binding of reactive metabolites to hepatic proteins, however, modifies the « self » of the subject. This may lead to immunization in a few subjects. The immune reaction may be directed either against the modified self (immunoallergy) or against the normal self (autoimmunity) (Figure 1).

Immunoallergic hepatitis : an immune reaction directed against protein or peptide epitopes modified by the covalent binding of reactive metabolites (reaction anti-modified self)

Many of the drugs transformed into reactive metabolites apparently lead to a type of hepatitis which is consistent with an immunological mechanism [1, 2]. Indeed, the liver injury is frequently associated with hypersensitivity manifestations, such as fever, blood eosinophilia, or other extrahepatic immunoallergic symptoms. Whereas hepatitis starts a few weeks to several months after the onset of the treatment during a first exposure to the drug, it may recur within a few hours or days during a second exposure. Immunoallergic hepatitis may be cytolytic, mixed or cholestatic [1, 2].

An example of immunoallergic hepatitis is the severe form of halothane-induced hepatitis. Halothane ($CF_3CHClBr$) is oxidatively metabolized by cytochrome P-450 into an unstable hydroxylated metabolite ($CF_3COHClBr$) which quickly looses HBr to form the reactive acyl chloride (CF_3COCl) [18]. This acylating intermediate reacts with the ϵ-NH_2 of lysine residues of proteins, to form CF_3CO-NH(lysine)-protein adducts [18]. Sera from patients with the severe form of halothane hepatitis contain antibodies which are directed against those parts of hepatic proteins which are modified by the covalent binding of the reactive halothane metabolite [19]. Trifluoroacetylated proteins include carboxylesterase, endoplasmin, calregulin, and protein disulfide isomerase [20]. It is not clear, however, whether these proteins (which are located in the endoplasmic reticulum lumen) can be expressed on the plasma membrane. Other, as yet unidentified, trifluoroacetylated proteins of the plasma membrane might serve as the actual antigenic targets.

Immune reactions against modified hepatic structures have also been reported in some cases of methyl dopa, tienilic acid and clometacin-induced hepatitis [references in 1].

A hypothethical mechanism [21] leading to immunization against modified protein or peptide epitopes is suggested in figure 2. While hepatocytes do not normally express major histocompatibility complex (MHC) class II molecules, these molecules are expressed on the surface of endothelial cells and Kupffer cells. During the cellular turnover of hepatocytes (particularly if this turnover is slightly increased by minor toxic effects of the drug), the cellular contents of dying hepatocytes will be engulfed by nearby macrophages (Figure 2). The phagocytized material will include proteins modified by the covalent binding of the reactive metabolite (« alkylated » proteins) (Figure 2). Macrophages will cut proteins into small peptidic fragments (including some « alkylated » peptides), and present some of these peptides (including the alkylated ones) in the groove of MHC class II molecules expressed on the cell surface (Figure 2).

While native, non-alkylated, peptides belong to the normal self of the individual, and should not be recognized by the T cell receptor (TCR) of circulating helper T cells, in contrast, alkylated peptides are different from the self, and may be recognized by the TCR of a few helper T cells (Figure 2). This may lead to the activation of these helper T cell clones.

Production of interleukin-2 by activated helper T cells may in turn stimulate the development of B cells producing antibodies against alkylated proteins, and the development of cytotoxic T cells (Figure 2). Antibodies against the modified self can recognize alkylated proteins (Figure 2), which are present on the hepatocyte plasma membrane [22, 23]. Cytotoxic T lymphocytes might recognize alkylated peptides presented by MHC class I molecules on the surface of hepatocytes [21] (Figure 2).

Autoimmune hepatitis : a reaction against the self triggered by the modified self

Autoantibodies with a high affinity for normal, non-alkylated, proteins have been recently described in a few forms of cytolytic drug-induced hepatitis [1]. Thus, in the serum of patients with tienilic acid-induced hepatitis, there are anti-liver/kidney microsome of type 2 (anti-LKM_2) autoantibodies [24]. These autoantibodies specifically recognize the particular isoenzyme of cytochrome P-450 (a member of the 2C subfamily) which transforms tienilic acid into a reactive metabolite which covalently binds to the cytochrome P-450 2C protein. Similarly, in the sera of subjects with dihydralazine hepatitis, there are antimicrosomal autoantibodies reacting with liver microsomes but not with kidney microsomes, and therefore termed « anti-LM » autoantibodies [25]. These autoantibodies specifically recognize cytochrome P-450 1A2, an isoenzyme which meta-

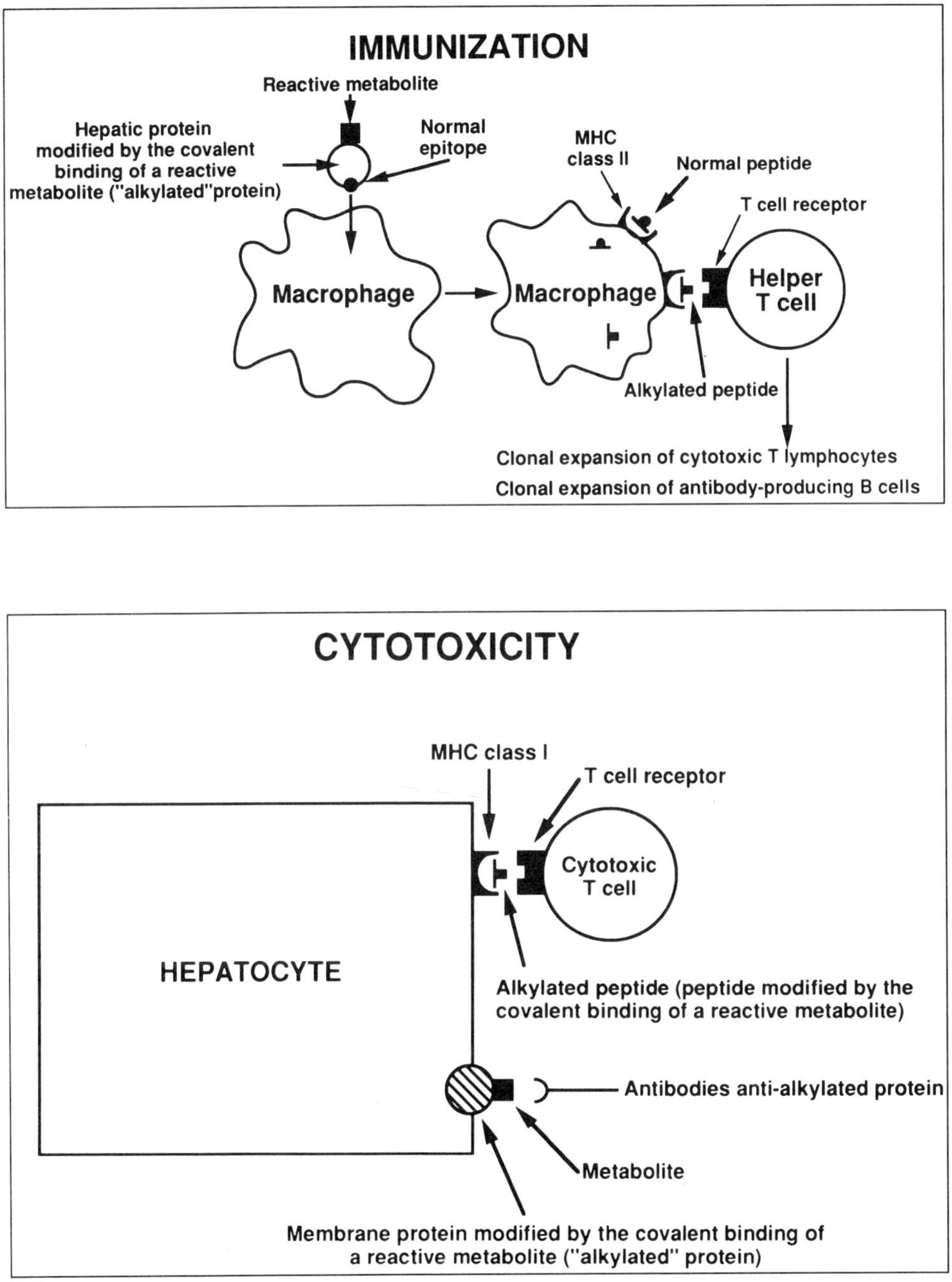

Figure 2. Hypothetical mechanisms for immunization against protein or peptide epitopes modified by the covalent binding of a reactive metabolite (reaction anti-modified self). See text for explanations.

bolizes dihydralazine into a reactive metabolite which then covalently binds to the cytochrome P-450 1A2 protein.

Both anti-LKM_2 and anti-LM autoantibodies recognize cytochromes P-450 from subjects not exposed to the drug. Thus, in both cases, the modification of self (due to covalent binding) leads to autoantibodies which recognize normal, unalkylated, epitopes of the protein.

A possible mechanism [21] is suggested in figure 3. Some B lymphocytes are autoreactive, but normally remain quiescent, since they are not stimulated by helper T cells. Let us consider an autoreactive B cell expressing a membrane immunoglobulin on its surface, which recognizes a normal (unalkylated) epitope of cytochrome P-450 1A2. After the death of a hepatocyte, this autoreactive B cell may capture a molecule of cytochrome P-450 1A2 by its normal epitope (Figure 3). If the subject has taken dihydralazine, the protein may be alkylated by the reactive metabolite on another part of the protein (Figure 3). After internalization and processing of the protein, the autoreactive B cell will present both nor-

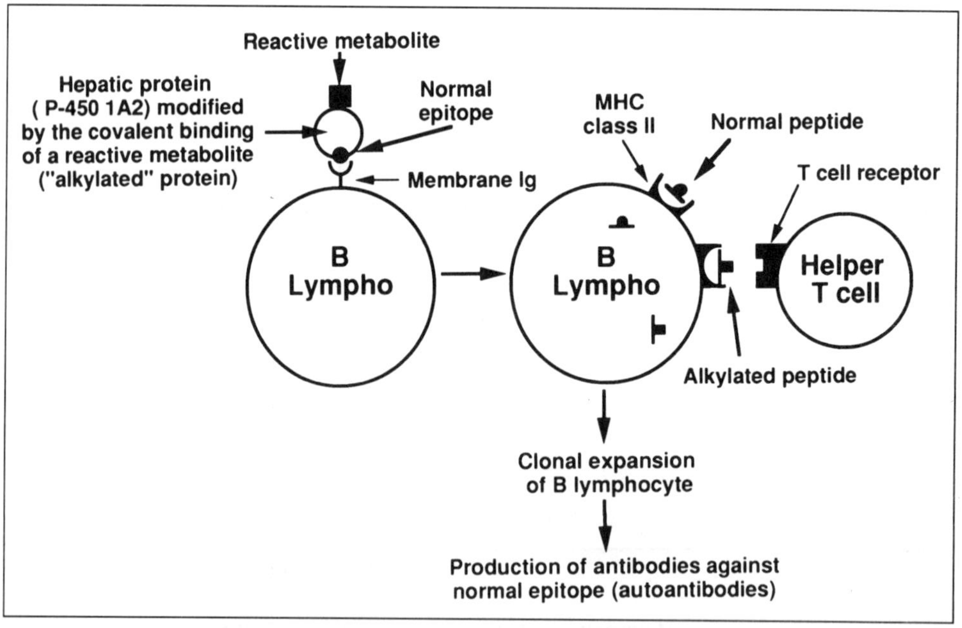

Figure 3. Hypothetical mechanisms for the appearance of autoantibodies directed against a normal protein epitope (reaction anti-self) after modification of another part of the molecule through the covalent binding of a reactive metabolite. See text for explanations.

mal peptides and alkylated peptides on its surface (on MHC class II molecules) (Figure 3). Normally, there are no helper T cells that will recognize normal peptides, which explains that the autoreactive B cell remains quiescent. In contrast, if an alkylated peptide is presented, some helper T cells may recognize this modified self (Figure 3). This recognition will lead to the clonal expansion and maturation of the autoreactive B lymphocyte that will secrete autoantibodies directed against the normal epitope of the hepatic protein (Figure 3). This hypothetical mechanism may explain an immunization against the self (autoantibodies), when another part of the protein has been modified by the covalent binding of a reactive metabolite (modified self) [21].

Several cytochromes P-450, including P-450 2C and 1A2, are present in the plasma membrane of human hepatocytes [26]. Some of the cytochrome P-450 epitopes recognized by anti-LKM_2 and anti-LM autoantibodies are expressed on the outer surface of the plasma membrane [26]. Thus, anti-cytochrome P-450 autoantibodies might participate (together with the probable involvement of cytotoxic T cells) in the immunological destruction of hepatocytes.

Probable coexistence of both autoantibodies and antibodies against altered self

In several patients with tienilic acid hepatitis, there were concomitantly anti-LKM_2 autoantibodies and antibodies recognizing tienilic acid-altered plasma membrane proteins, suggesting that immunization in this type of hepatitis may be directed both against the normal self and against the modified self [27]. It is tempting to speculate that such a dual immunization might also occur in other forms of hepatitis due to immune mechanisms.

Genetic factors involved in immune hepatitis

Although all subjects probably form the reactive metabolite to some extent, only a few develop immunization and hepatitis. Two types of genetic factors may intervene in the unique susceptibility of these subjects. Whereas alkylation of a few molecules of hepatic proteins might lead to uncommon immunization, more extensive alkylation of hepatic proteins might lead to more frequent immunization. This might occur, for example, if some subjects are deficient in inactivating mechanism(s) [28]. Defects in protective mechanisms have been suggested as risk factors in immunoallergic hepatitis due to phenytoin, carbamazepine, phenobarbital, sulphonamide, amineptine, and possibly also halothane [references in 29]. The deficit(s) involved remain unknown.

A second type of genetic factor is the MHC phenotype, also termed the human leukocyte antigen (HLA) phenotype in humans. Different HLA molecules may present different peptides. It is therefore possible that some HLA class I or II molecules may permit the presentation of some alkylated peptides [1]. Indeed, one particular HLA molecule seems to favour hepatitis due to some drugs, while other HLA molecules favour hepatitis due to other drugs [references in 30].

Granulomatous hepatitis

Small rounded foci of epithelioid cells and round cells (with sometimes multinucleated giant cells) are found in the portal tracts or hepatic lobule [2]. Such granulomas strongly suggest an allergic mechanism [1]. Little is known, however, of the specific mechanism(s) leading to this lesion.

Acute bland cholestasis

In this condition, the only liver lesion is cholestasis, without inflammation or necrosis. Acute bland cholestasis is apparently due to an interference with bile secretion. Oestrogens interfere with bile secretion through three mechanisms [references in 1]. *a)* Prolonged administration of oestrogens increases the permeability of the paracellular pathway, leading to back-diffusion of materials from bile canaliculi to blood. *b)* Prolonged administration of oestrogens produces increased activity of cholesterol acylCoA transferase and leads to the accumulation of cholesterol esters in plasma membrane ; this may decrease membrane fluidity and inhibit Na^+, K^+-ATPase activity. *c)* Finally, oestrogens are quickly transformed into D-ring (17-β) glucuronides which exhibit an immediate and extremely potent cholestatic effect. Although these effects may be observed at high doses in all subjects, some women have a genetically determined susceptibility to these cholestatic effects.

Anabolic/androgenic steroids with a C-17 alkyl substituent also interfere with bile secretion by inhibiting Na^+, K^+-ATPase (an effect which may reduce bile acid uptake) and by altering the pericanalicular microfilamentous network (which may impair contractions of bile canaliculi) [references in 1].

Steatosis

Although there are transitions between these forms, it is convenient to distinguish two types of steatosis : macrovacuolar and microvesicular steatosis.

Macrovacuolar steatosis

In this type of steatosis, the hepatocyte contains a single, large, fat droplet which displaces the nucleus to the periphery of the cell [2]. An impaired egress of lipids from the liver is thought to be the main mechanism for this lesion [30]. Triglycerides leave the liver in the form of lipoproteins. Their apoprotein moieties are glycoproteins which are synthesized in the rough endoplasmic reticulum and are glycolysated both there and in the Golgi apparatus. The decreased output of triglycerides may be a result of a specific biochemical lesion, as with methotrexate which impairs protein synthesis. It may also occur due to structural lesions of the endoplasmic reticulum, Golgi apparatus and plasma membrane, which explains why macrovacuolar steatosis is sometimes associated with hepatitis produced by many drugs (such as allopurinol, halothane, isoniazid, and α-methyldopa).

Microvesicular steatosis

In this condition, numerous small lipid vesicules occupy the hepatocyte, leaving the nucleus in the centre of the cell. Liver cell necrosis may be absent (as with tetracycline) or present (as with valproic acid) [2]. Even without cell necrosis, extensive microvesicular steatosis is a serious condition, which may lead to liver failure, coma and death [2]. Microvesicular steatosis is related to the inhibition of the mitochondrial oxidation of fatty acids [1]. When poorly oxidized in mitochondria, fatty acids undergo increased esterification into triglycerides, which accumulate as small lipid vesicules in the liver. The impairment of mitochondrial function and energy production may perhaps explain the hepatic insufficiency and poor prognosis which is characteristic of severe forms of microvesicular steatosis. Decreased β-oxidation of fatty acids has been demonstrated with valproic acid, pirprofen, ibuprofen, amineptine, amiodarone, tetracycline, and several tetracycline derivatives [references in 31]. Similarly, several Reye-like syndromes are caused by various constitutive defects in mitochondrial β-oxidation enzymes, and Reye's syndrome itself is due to an acquired mitochondrial dysfunction [1]. Cytokines, such as tumor necrosis factor or interferon, may be involved by decreasing the expression of mitochondrial genes and mitochondrial respiration [references in 1]. Salicylic acid potentiates the occurrence of Reye's syndrome by inhibiting the activation and thus β-oxidation of long chain fatty acids [32], thus aggravating a mitochondrial function already hampered by post-infectious factors.

Phospholipidosis and alcoholic-like liver lesions

These lesions are mainly seen with the three antianginal drugs diethylaminoethoxyhexestrol, perhexiline maleate, and amiodarone [2]. These drugs are cationic amphiphilic compounds with a lipophilic moiety and an ionizeable nitrogen (which becomes positively charged).

The uncharged molecule may enter lysosomes, where the drug may then be trapped, in its protonated form, due to the acidic intralysosomal milieu [1]. The amphiphilic drug which accumulates within lysosomes may form a stable complex with phospholipids, and inhibit the action of intralysosomal phospholipases [33]. Phospholipids which are not degraded, progressively accumulate, along with the drug, in lysosomes. Lysosomes are increased in size, and contain pseudo-myelinic figures.

The same amphiphilic characteristics may explain pseudo-alcoholic liver lesions [34, 35 and still unpublished observations from our laboratory]. Electron transfer along the mitochondrial respiratory chain is associated with the extrusion of protons from the mitochondrial matrix to the intermembranous space of the mitochondrion, creating a large membrane potential across the inner mitochondrial membrane (Figure 4). The protonated drug (amiodarone, perhexiline or diethylaminoethoxyhexestrol) enters the mitochondria along this membrane potential, reaches high intramitochondrial concentrations, and inhibits both the respiratory chain (leading to decreased ATP formation and liver cell necrosis) and β-oxidation enzymes (leading to steatosis) (Figure 4). Steatosis may in turn lead to lipid peroxidation [36], which releases chemoattractants (responsible for polymorphonuclear cell infiltration) and malondialdehyde (a bifunctional aldehyde, which might cross-link cytokeratins, and lead to Mallory bodies formation) (Figure 4).

Perhexiline maleate is transformed into hydroxylated metabolites which are eliminated. This transformation is mediated by the isoenzyme of cytochrome P-450 (P-450 2D6) which metabolizes debrisoquine, sparteine, dextromethorphan, and several other drugs. This isoenzyme is deficient in 3 to 10 per cent of Caucasians. In these subjects, perhexiline maleate is poorly oxidized and accumulates to a greater extent. These subjects are uniquely susceptible to the development of perhexiline maleate-induced neuropathy and liver disease [37].

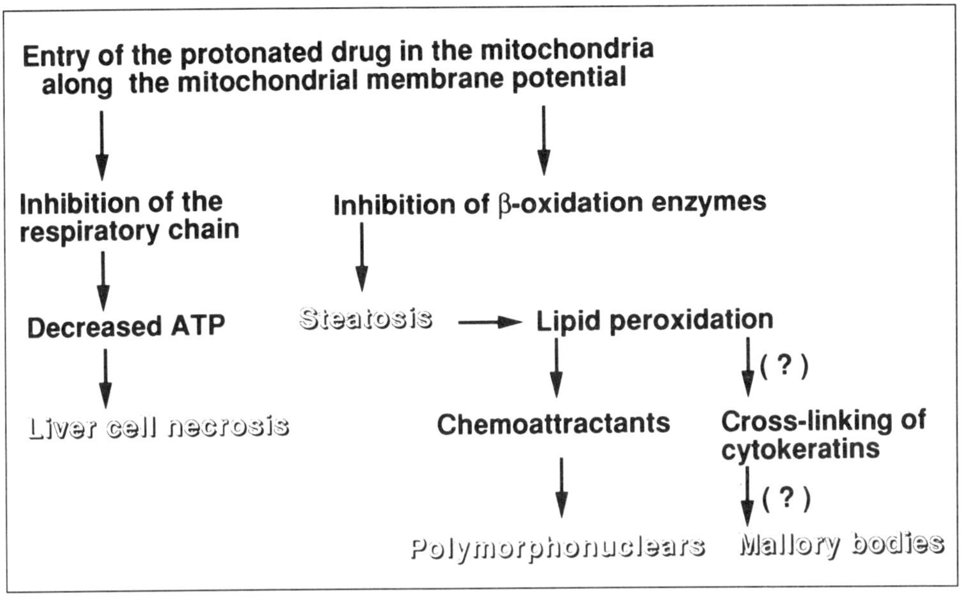

Figure 4. Possible mechanisms of alcoholic-like liver lesions. See text for explanations.

Outlook

Over the past 15 years, considerable progress has been made in unravelling the mechanisms whereby drugs produce various liver lesions. Several concepts have been proposed, and a major mechanism is now apparent for each liver lesion.

It is clear, however, that the present understanding represents, at best, a simplified overview of reality. Because there are so many hepatotoxic drugs, only a few aspects, if any, have been investigated for any single drug. As other aspects are explored, other hepatotoxic mechanisms will probably be disclosed. Like ethanol, which (though a very simple molecule) produces a variety of deleterious effects on the liver, some drugs (which are usually much more complex molecules) may be hepatotoxic through a variety of different mechanisms.

References

1. Pessayre D. Mechanisms of drug-induced hepatic injury. In : Stricker BHC, ed. Drug-induced hepatic injury, second edition. Amsterdam : Elsevier, 1992 : 23-49.
2. Pessayre D, Larrey D. Drug-induced liver injury. In : McIntyre N, Benhamou JP, Bircher J, Rizzetto M, Rodés J, eds. Oxford textbook of clinical hepatology, volume 2. Oxford : Oxford University Press, 1991 : 875-902.
3. Gonzales FJ, Nebert DW. Evolution of the cytochrome P-450 gene superfamily : animal-plant « warfare », molecular drive and human genetic differences in drug oxidation. Trends Genet 1990 ; 6 : 182-6.
4. Guengerich FP, Liebler DC. Enzymatic activation of chemicals to toxic metabolites. CRC Crit Rev Toxicol 1985 ; 14 : 259-307.
5. Mirabelli F, Salis A, Marinoni V, *et al.* Menadione-induced bleb formation in hepatocytes is associated with the oxidation of thiol groups in actin. Arch Biochem Biophys 1988 ; 264 : 261-9.
6. Fagian MM, Pereira-Da-Silva L, Martins IS, Vercesi AE. Membrane protein thiol cross-linking associated with the permeabilization of the inner membrane by Ca^{2+} plus prooxidants. J Biol Chem 1990 ; 265 : 19955-60.
7. Nicotera P, Bellomo G, Orrenius S. Calcium-mediated mechanisms in chemically induced cell death. Annu Rev Pharmacol Toxicol 1992 ; 32 : 449-70.
8. Larrey D, Lettéron P, Foliot A, *et al.* Effects of pregnancy on the toxicity and metabolism of acetaminophen in mice. J Pharmacol Exp Ther 1986 ; 237 : 283-91.
9. Pessayre D, Dolder A, Artigou JY, *et al.* Effect of fasting on metabolite-mediated hepatotoxicity in the rat. Gastroenterology 1979 ; 77 : 264-71.
10. Pessayre D, Bentata M, Degott C, *et al.* Isoniazid-rifampin fulminant hepatitis. A possible consequence of the enhancement of isoniazid hepatotoxicity by enzyme induction. Gastroenterology 1977 ; 72 : 284-9.
11. Pessayre D, de Saint-Louvent P, Degott C, Bernuau J, Rueff B, Benhamou JP. Iproclozide fulminant hepatitis. Possible role of enzyme induction. Gastroenterology 1978 ; 75 : 492-6.
12. Seef LB, Cucherini BA, Zimmerman HJ, Adler E, Benjamin SB. Acetaminophen hepatotoxicity in alcoholics. A therapeutic misadventure. Ann Intern Med 1986 ; 104 : 399-404.
13. Shaw S, Rubin KP, Lieber CS. Depressed hepatic glutathione and increased diene conjugates in alcoholic liver disease. Evidence of lipid peroxidation. Dig Dis Sci 1983 ; 28 : 585-9.
14. Pessayre D, Wandscheer JC, Cobert B, *et al.* Additive effects of inducers and fasting on acetaminophen hepatotoxicity. Biochem Pharmacol 1980 ; 29 : 2219-23.
15. Jacqz E, Hall SD, Branch RA. Genetically determined polymorphisms in drug oxidation. Hepatology 1986 ; 6 : 1020-32.
16. Larrey D, Tinel M, Amouyal G, *et al.* Genetically determined oxidation polymorphism and drug hepatotoxicity. Study of 51 patients. J Hepatol 1989, 8 : 158-64.
17. Spielberg SP, Gordon GB. Glutathione synthetase-deficient lymphocytes and acetaminophen toxicity. Clin Pharmacol Ther 1981 ; 29 : 51-5.
18. Sipes IG, Gandolfi J, Pohl LR, Krishna G, Brown BR. Comparison of the biotransformation and hepatotoxicity of halothane and deuterated halothane. J Pharmacol Exp Ther 1980 ; 214 : 716-20.
19. Kenna JG, Satoh H, Christ DD, Pohl LR. Metabolic basis for a drug hypersensitivity : antibodies in sera from patients with halothane hepatitis recognize liver neoantigens that contain the trifluoacetyl group derived from halothane. J Pharmacol Exp Ther 1988 ; 245 : 1103-9.
20. Pohl LR. Drug-induced allergic hepatitis. Semin Liver Dis 1990 ; 10 : 305-15.
21. Pessayre D. Physiopathologie des hépatopathies médicamenteuses. Gastroenterol Clin Biol (in press).
22. Loeper J, Descatoire V, Amouyal G, Lettéron P, Larrey D, Pessayre D. Presence of covalently bound metabolites on rat hepatocyte plasma membrane proteins after admi-

nistration of isaxonine, a drug leading to immunoallergic hepatitis in man. Hepatology 1989 ; 9 : 675-8.
23. Satoh H, Fukuda Y, Anderson DK, Ferrans VJ, Gillette JR, Pohl LR. Immunological studies on the mechanism of halothane-induced hepatotoxicity : immunohistochemical evidence of trifluoroacetylated hepatocytes. J Pharmacol Exp Ther 1985 ; 233 : 857-62.
24. Beaune P, Dansette PM, Mansuy D, *et al.* Human anti-endoplasmic reticulum autoantibodies appearing in a drug-induced hepatitis are directed against a human liver cytochrome P-450 that hydrolates the drug. Proc Natl Acad Sci USA 1987 ; 84 : 551-5.
25. Bourdi M, Larrey D, Nataf J, *et al.* Anti-liver endoplasmic reticulum autoantibodies are directed against human liver cytochrome P-450 IA2. A specific marker of dihydralazine-induced hepatitis. J Clin Invest 1990 ; 85 : 1967-73.
26. Loeper J, Descatoire V, Maurice M, *et al.* Cytochrome P-450 in human hepatocyte plasma membrane : recognition by several autoantibodies. Gastroenterology 1993 ; 104 : 203-16.
27. Neuberger J, Williams R. Immune mechanisms in tienilic acid associated hepatotoxicity. Gut 1989 ; 30 : 515-9.
28. Larrey D, Berson A, Habersetzer F, *et al.* Genetic predisposition to drug hepatotoxicity. Role in hepatitis caused by amineptine, a tricyclic antidepressant. Hepatology 1989 ; 10 : 168-73.
29. Berson A, Fréneaux E, Larrey D, *et al.* Possible role of the HLA haplotype in hepatotoxicity. An exploratory study in 71 patients with drug-induced idiosyncratic hepatitis. J Hepatol (in press).
30. Zimmerman HJ. Hepatotoxicity. The adverse effects of drugs and other chemicals on the liver. New York : Appleton Century Crofts, 1978.
31. Grimbert S, Fromenty B, Fisch C, *et al.* Decreased mitochondrial oxidation of fatty acids in pregnant mice. Possible relevance to the development of acute fatty liver of pregnancy. Hepatology (in press).
32. Deschamps D, Fisch C, Fromenty B, Berson A, Degott C, Pessayre D. Inhibition by salicylic acid of the activation and thus oxidation of long chain fatty acids. Possible role in the development of Reye's syndrome. J Pharmacol Exp Ther 1991 ; 259 : 894-904.
33. Kubo M, Hostetler KY. Diethylaminoethoxyhexestrol inhibition of purified rat liver lysosomal phospholipase A1 : role of drug binding to substrate. J Pharmacol Exp Ther 1986 ; 240 : 88-92.
34. Fromenty B, Fisch C, Labbe G, *et al.* Amiodarone inhibits the mitochondrial β-oxidation of fatty acids and produces microvesicular steatosis of the liver in mice. J Pharmacol Exp Ther 1990 ; 255 : 1371-6.
35. Fromenty B, Fisch C, Berson A, Lettéron P, Larrey D, Pessayre D. Dual effect of amiodarone on mitochondrial respiration. Initial protonophoric uncoupling effect followed by inhibition of the respiratory chain at the levels of complex I and complex II. J Pharmacol Exp Ther 1990 ; 255 : 1377-84.
36. Lettéron P, Duchatelle V, Berson A, *et al.* Increased ethane exhalation, an *in vivo* index of lipid peroxidation, in alcohol-abusers. Gut 1993 ; 34 : 409-14.
37. Morgan MY, Reshef R, Shah RR, Oates NS, Smith RL, Sherlock S. Impaired oxidation of debrisoquine in patients with perhexiline liver injury. Gut 1984 ; 10 : 1057-64.

Progress in Hepatology 93. J.P. Miguet and D. Dhumeaux, eds.
John Libbey Eurotext, Paris © 1993, pp. 41-46

4

Pathobiology of hepatitis B virus infection and mechanism of action of interferon

A. ALBERTI

Clinica Medica II°, University of Padova, 35126 Padova, Italy.

To understand how interferon (IFN) -alpha may act as a therapeutic agent for chronic hepatitis B, it is essential to consider first the pathogenesis of liver damage and of virus clearance occurring in the natural course of the disease as IFN is most likely to produce its effects by acting upon these pathways.

The hepatitis B virus (HBV) is a double-stranded DNA agent which causes a wide spectrum of clinical manifestations in the infected host, including fulminant liver damage, asymptomatic and self-limited acute infection, chronic infection with progressive liver disease and a healthy chronic carrier state.

The virus is not thought to be directly cytopathic [1] and the determinants of such different clinical outcomes have been only partially understood, being identified in : *a)* the repertoire of host immune response to the virus and *b)*, more recently, the existence of genomic variants of HBV, the two being closely interwoven.

The interaction of HBV with the infected host implies several events of pathogenetic importance each of which has been extensively studied in recent years : *a)* attachment of HBV to hepatocytes through specific receptors, *b)* replication of HBV in the cell with synthesis and processing of viral proteins some of which become expressed on the surface of infected hepatocytes, *c)* a complex network of immune response to the virus, including T and B cell responses which become involved in causing liver damage, in controlling virus replication, in clearing the virus infection, but also in generating escape mutants of the virus.

Attachment of HBV to hepatocytes and the intracellular replicative cycle

Envelope proteins of HBV mediate its attachment to hepatocytes [2]. We and others have shown that the preS1 domain of the large envelope protein of HBV is critical for binding which seems to occur by interaction with hepatocyte membrane receptors for physiological ligands. Indeed, it has been proposed that HBV may use IgA receptors or receptors for asyaloglycoproteins, interleukin-6 or transferrin, but definitive clarification of this issue has not yet been achieved.

Replication of HBV in liver cells occurs through four major steps [3] : *a)* conversion of asymmetric virion DNA to covalently closed circular DNA, *b)* transcription of this DNA to produce a pregenome RNA template for reverse transcription, *c)* encapsidation of the pregenome into virus cases and synthesis of minus-stranded DNA, *d)* synthesis of the plus-strand.

This replication pathway implies that viral RNA serves as both template for genomic DNA and messenger RNA for synthesis of viral proteins.

Among the viral proteins encoded by HBV, those which become expressed on the surface of virion and/or of hepatocytes are more likely to be involved in pathogenesis. The envelope proteins generate virus neutralizing antibodies. They have been also localized on the surface of infected cells where they can act as targets for cytotoxic reactions [4]. However, the nucleocapsid proteins (HBcAg and HBeAg) are thought to be the major targets of the immune responses responsible for the lysis of infected cells supporting virus activity. It is unclear whether HBcAg or HBeAg, or both, are exposed on infected hepatocytes. Killing by cytotoxic T cells would probably occur anyway because HBcAg and HBeAg T cell epitopes may be presented in the form of identical partial peptides which have been processed inside the cell. Other studies, however, have shown that HBeAg but not HBcAg epitopes can be recognized on liver cells by antibody dependent cytotoxic reactions [5].

Immune response to HBV antigens and pathogenesis of liver damage and of HBV clearance

The vast majority of non-immunocompromised patients who acquire HBV infection recover with clearance of the virus. The determinants of recovery are not fully understood and may include : *a)* production of interferons which generate an antiviral state in the liver, reduce virus replication and induce MHC class I glycoprotein expression on infected hepatocytes, *b)* NK cell activation, *c)* later generation of virus-specific cytotoxic T cell, *d)* intrahepatic production and release of cytokines, such as interleukins, interferon-gamma, tumor necrosis factor (TNF) -alpha, etc. which may directly contribute to killing of infected and uninfected hepatocytes, *e)* production of antiviral antibodies with neutralizing activity which act by limiting the reinfection of liver cells by circulating virions. The concerted action of these mechanisms leads to recovery while defects may cause chronicity. If the defect is only a partial one, it can be overcome either spontaneously during transient rebound of immunocompetence or with the administration of immunopotentiators or/of interferon ; while if it is more profound and stable it is highly unlikely that it might be corrected. This latter situation is that typically occurring in neonates born to HBeAg positive carrier mothers [6]. They become completely tolerant to nucleocapsid proteins due to specific unresponsiveness of helper T cells to HBcAg and to HBeAg caused by soluble HBeAg transferred from mother's blood to the fetus. These children usually have little evidence of liver damage and do not respond to interferon therapy.

There is no doubt that the T cell response to endogenously synthetized HBV proteins which become expressed with HLA class I antigens on the surface of infected hepatocytes represents the major determinant of the lysis of infected cells and, when this mechanism is fully efficient, of recovery from infection. Most relevant data to understand such events have come in recent years from the excellent work of Ferrari and of his colleagues [7].

Extensive research carried out in Chisari's laboratory in La Jolla, California, and then at the University of Parma, in Italy, has led to the demonstration that patients who recover from hepatitis B develop HLA class I restricted T cell cytotoxicity against HBV infected cells. Cytotoxic T cells recognize a short cytotoxic T lymphocyte (CTL) epitope which is included within the 11-27 sequence of the core antigen and is shared with the e antigen. Recognition of the epitope by peripheral lymphocytes of patients with chronic infection is less efficient than in subjects who clear the virus, suggesting that absent or weak response to core could be the defect responsible for chronicity. It remains to be clarified whether this HLA restricted cytotoxicity is involved in causing liver damage in chronic hepatitis B. Ehata *et al.* [8] found that chronic HBV carriers with progressive liver disease often have mutations of a small segment of the core antigen while carriers without liver disease have not such changes suggesting that this sequence contains a major target of CTL and that the mutations evolve under the pressure of immune selection. Beside nucleocapsid antigens, envelope antigens may also be involved as CTL targets, as shown for preS2 [9] and for HBsAg. Furthermore, killing of HBsAg containing hepatocytes as well as of normal bystander cells may also occur as a consequence of direct cytotoxicity by cytokines (particularly IFN-gamma and TNF-alpha) released in the liver during immunoreactive events [10].

Mechanism of action of interferon in chronic hepatitis B

The rationale for treating patients with chronic hepatitis B with IFN-alpha lies in the observation that they have a reduced capacity to produce endogenous IFN [11].

It has also been shown that HBV itself specifically reduces the capacity of the cells that it infects to respond to IFN, but such refractoriness to IFN may be overcome by increasing concentrations of IFN. The first effect seen in chronic hepatitis B after administration of IFN-alpha is an immediate fall in serum HBV-DNA levels, most likely as a consequence of direct antiviral effects [12]. It may reflect inhibition in the processing or transport of virus glycoproteins or other effects on maturation and release of virus particles, but the major antiviral effects seem those caused by the ds- RNA dependent 2,5A synthetase and protein kinase system which affect mainly the synthesis of viral proteins [13]. Suppression of HBV replication may be the only effect of interferon therapy and in such cases there is usually only a transient response to treatment and virus replication starts again soon after cessation of IFN administration.

In other patients, and typically in those who become permanent responders with HBeAg to anti-HBe seroconversion and definitive loss of HBV replication, a sharp rise in serum transaminase levels is observed after 5 to 8 weeks of therapy. This hepatitis « flare » most likely reflects enhancement of the immune mediated lysis of infected (and uninfected ?) liver cells.

The delay in appearance of the ALT peak during therapy favours the hypothesis of recruitment of cytotoxic T rather than NK cells and may be due to the need of reaching, by the direct antiviral effect, a significant reduction in levels of circulating virions and viral antigens which would otherwise « paralize » cytotoxic T cells. Interferon-alpha most likely promotes the ALT flare by optimizing the presentation of viral antigens at the hepatocyte surface to CTLs. This effect may be mediated by enhancement of class I MCH glycoproteins expression in the presence of already activated antigen specific cytotoxic T cells. On the other hand, IFN-alpha is most likely ineffective in the absence of activated T cells and would not favour activation of resting T cells. This explains why patients who respond to IFN therapy are those with pretreatment more active disease and most likely to undergo spontaneous anti-HBe seroconversion and loss of HBV replication, if left untreated. Thus IFN therapy seems to act by potentiating the natural pathway of the individual response against infected hepatocytes and it may be therefore inferred that it may occasionally favour the selection of virus escape mutants, and this may cause failure of treatment.

Although it was reported that higher degree of HLA class I display on hepatocytes correlates with successful response to IFN, some authors have suggested that HLA class II display may also have a role [14]. However, IFN-alpha is not as good as IFN-gamma in inducing HLA class II antigens and recent data [15] correlating ALT levels, HLA class I antigens display on hepatocytes, serum beta2 microglobulin levels and intrahepatic $CD8^+$ cells seem to support the hypothesis that IFN potentiates HLA-restricted $CD8^+$ cells cytotoxicity.

It remains to be explored how the administration of exogenous IFN-alpha could affect the destruction of HBsAg positive hepatocytes mediated by IFN-gamma and by other cytokines, a mechanism that has been recently proposed as a possible cause of liver cell damage in chronic HBV infection. IFN-alpha therapy promotes the production of IFN-gamma and of TNF- alpha [16] and these cytokines may amplify the destruction of liver cells by acting on HBsAg positive and, possibly, on HBsAg negative (bystanders) hepatocytes. These effects may lead to severe liver cell necrosis in the presence of large number of HBsAg positive cells, but this mechanism could also explain the disappearance of HBsAg positive cells with integrated HBV genome that may occur in chronic HBsAg carriers who become HBsAg negative with IFN therapy.

References

1. Alberti A, Tremolada F, Fattovich G, Bortolotti F, Realdi G. Virus replication and liver disease in chronic hepatitis B virus infection. Dig Dis Sci 1983 ; 28 : 962-6.
2. Alberti A, Gerlich WH, Hlermann KH, Pontisso P. Nature and display of hepatitis B virus envelope proteins and the humoral immune response. Springer Semin Immunopathol 1990 ; 12 : 5-23.
3. Ganem D, Karmus HE. The molecular biology of the hepatitis B viruses. Annu Rev Biochem 1987 ; 56 : 651-93.
4. Alberti A, Realdi G, Tremolada F, Cadrobbi P. HBsAg on liver cell surface in viral hepatitis. Lancet 1975 ; 1 : 346.
5. Schlicht H, Von Brunn A, Theilmann L. Antibodies in anti-HBe positive patient sera bind to an HBe protein expressed on the cell surface of human hepatoma cells : implications for virus clearance. Hepatology 1991 ; 13 : 57-61.
6. Milich DR, Jones JE, Hughes JL, Price J, Roney AK, McLachlan A. Is a function of the secreted hepatitis e antigen to induce immunologic tolerance *in utero* ? Proc Natl Acad Sci USA 1990 ; 87 : 6588-608.
7. Penna A, Chisari FV, Bertoletti A, Missale G, Fowler P, Giuberti T, Fiaccadori F, Ferrari C. Cytotoxic T lymphocytes recognize an HLA-A2 restricted epitope within the hepatitis B virus nucleocapside antigen. J Exp Med 1991 ; 174 : 1565-70.
8. Ehata T, Omata M, Yokosuka O, Hosoda K, Ohto M. Variations in codons 84-101 in the core nucleotide sequence correlate with hepatocellular injury in chronic hepatitis B virus infection. J Clin Invest 1992 ; 89 : 332-8.
9. Barnaba V, Franco A, Alberti A, Balsano C, Benvenuto R, Balsano F. Recognition of hepatitis B virus envelope proteins by liver infiltrating T lymphocytes in chronic HBV infection. J Immunol 1989 ; 143 : 2650-5.
10. Gilles PN, Guerrette DL, Ulevitch RJ, Schreiber D, Chisari FV. HBsAg retention sensitises the hepatocyte to injury by physiological concentrations of interferon-gamma. Hepatology 1992 ; 16 : 655-63.
11. Thomas HC. Pathogenesis of chronic HBV infection and mechanisms of action of antiviral compounds. In : Hollinger FB, Lemon SM, Morgolis HS, eds. Viral hepatitis and liver disease. Baltimore : Williams and Wilkins, 1991 : 612-5.
12. Kerr IM, Slark GR. The antiviral effects of the interferons and their inhibition. J Interferon Res 1992 ; 12 : 237-40.
13. Peters M. Mechanisms of action of interferons. Semin Liver Dis 1989 ; 9 : 235-9.
14. Paul RG, Roodman ST, Campbell GR, Bodickly C, Perillo RP. HLA class I antigen expression as a measure of response to antiviral therapy of chronic hepatitis B. Hepatology 1991 ; 13 : 820-5.
15. Hayata T, Nakano Y, Yoshisawa K, Sodeyama T, Kiyosawa K. Effects of interferon on intrahepatic human leukocyte antigens and lymphocyte subsets in patients with chronic hepatitis B and C. Hepatology 1991 ; 13 : 1022-8.
16. Daniels HM, Meager A, Eddleston ALW, Alexander GJM, Williams R. Spontaneous production of tumor necrosis factor alpha and interleukin-1 beta during interferon-alpha treatment of chronic HBV infection. Lancet 1990 ; 335 : 875-7.

Progress in Hepatology 93. J.P. Miguet and D. Dhumeaux, eds.
John Libbey Eurotext, Paris © 1993, pp. 47-53

5

Long-term follow-up of interferon responders in chronic hepatitis B

R.P. PERRILLO, A.L. MASON

Gastroenterology Section, Veterans Affairs Medical Center and Washington University School of Medicine, Saint Louis, MO 63106, USA.

A response to alpha interferon occurs in approximately 40 % of patients with chronic hepatitis B [1-3]. This has generally been defined as the disappearance of hepatitis B e antigen (HBeAg) and HBV DNA in serum as evaluated by dot blot or solution hybridization [1, 4]. The loss of these circulating markers of viral replication is either associated with a major reduction or normalization in aminotransferase levels and improvement in liver histology, including diminished piecemeal necrosis and portal inflammatory infiltration [2, 5]. The majority of the published literature, however, is based upon short-term (6 to 12 months) posttreatment follow-up, and less is known about the more remote effects of therapy. A number of studies have recently emphasized the long-term benefits of therapy from both virological and clinical perspectives [6-13]. It is the purpose of this paper to briefly review recent studies in these areas, with special reference to observations derived after the first year of follow-up.

Delayed clearance of HBeAg

The conventional definition of a response to interferon therapy has come to mean the sustained loss of HBeAg and HBV DNA. In approximately 10 % of treated individuals in the US multicenter trial of interferon alpha, however, a sustained loss of HBV DNA occurred that was not associated with immediate HBeAg clearance [1]. In that study, patients reaching this endpoint were termed « indeterminate responders ». This term belies the importance of this result, however, because biochemical and histological improvement was documented in these patients [2]. Moreover, several of the indeterminate responders exhibited delayed clearance of HBeAg during the second year of posttreatment observation (R. Perrillo, unpublished data). Similar observations have been made by Lok and colleagues in a recent study involving 128 Asian HBV carriers [11]. In that study, delayed clearance of HBeAg occurred in 28 (22 %) of patients who had been treated with interferon alpha, either alone or following prednisone withdrawal. Delayed clearance of HBeAg occurred more often in HBeAg positive patients who remained serum HBV DNA negative by direct spot hybridization after treatment when compared to those who remained HBV DNA positive (6 of 11 or 55 % *vs* 22 of 88 or 25 %). All six patients who remained HBV DNA negative at the end of a 6 month posttreatment follow-up cleared their HBeAg within the second year. These studies indicate that delayed clearance of HBeAg, usually within the second year, is not uncommon in both Caucasian and Asian patients who remain HBV DNA negative after therapy.

Frequency of relapse

In the United States and Western Europe, between 5 % to 10 % of responders will relapse within the first year after therapy [2, 7]. Several studies have demonstrated that the disappearance of markers of viral replication tends to be maintained indefinitely in patients who remain HBV DNA negative during the first 12 to 18 months of follow-up [3, 7, 14]. Both features have been nicely demonstrated in a study conducted by Korenman and associates at the National Institutes of Health [7]. In that study, 3 of 23 responders (13 %) relapsed within the first year after therapy. Responses were maintained in the remaining 20 patients during a follow-up period that spanned 3 to 7 years. Of note, one of the 3 patients who relapsed early developed HIV-related lymphadenopathy syndrome shortly after deterioration of hepatitis B. This is similar to the data of Krogsgaard and colleagues who suggested that HIV-1 infected patients may reactivate their hepatitis more frequently [15]. The frequency of early and late relapse is probably also higher in Asian HBV carriers. In the Lok study, for example, 7 responders (24 %) reactivated, with the majority (5 % or 17 %) doing this in the second posttreatment year. Late relapse occurred in 2 patients (7 %), however, at 3.5 and 5 years. Another group that has been observed to relapse more frequently are patients infected with a precore mutant virus [16, 17].

Histological assessment

Histological improvement appears to be maintained in responders during prolonged follow-up [9, 10]. My colleagues and I have recently described our results in patients in a small group of patients in whom HBsAg disappeared [9]. In that study, 7 patients (5 of whom had been treated) were blindly evaluated by the Knodell criteria at intervals that ranged from 3 months to 67 months after HBsAg clearance and 26 months to 87 months after HBeAg clearance. The degree of histological improvement was most marked 4 or more years after the disappearance of HBeAg and HBsAg ; in some instances it was difficult to distinguish any histological abnormality (total Knodell scores of 0 to 1). In a similar study conducted at the National Institutes of Health [10] patients were evaluated at intervals varying from 0.6 to 9 years after loss of HBsAg. A mild degree of « septal hepatitis » was observed in many of these patients, even at the most remote timepoints. Nonetheless, this study also affirmed a marked overall improvement when compared to baseline biopsies. It appears from these studies that histological restitution occurs slowly and may not always be complete, even when liver biopsy is done years after the loss of HBsAg. However, the degree of residual inflammation is usually slight and the improvement is much greater than that observed in short-term histological assessments.

Recently, we have had the opportunity to histologically evaluate a group of patients who remained HBsAg positive but HBeAg negative years after a response was achieved. Multiple posttreatment biopsies were available in some instances. As can be seen in Table I, the histological appearance of biopsies obtained a few months after the disappearance of HBV DNA and HBeAg was not always interpreted as improved when compared to baseline assessments (patients 5 and 6). The same individuals, however, demonstrated marked resolution of inflammation in biopsies obtained approximately 2.8 and 4.4 years, respectively, after a response was achieved. These data, therefore, are reminiscent of the findings described above in patients in whom the HBsAg marker disappeared.

Virological status

A number of investigators have assessed whether HBV infection is totally eradicated in patients who become HBsAg negative as a result of

Table I. Clinical, serological, and histological features of long-term HBeAg/HBV DNA negative patients : Washington University Experience.

	Age (years)	Duration (in years) of Neg HBeAg	Duration (in years) of Normal ALT	Biopsy report Initial	Biopsy report Follow-up
1.	63	.75	.60	CAH, possible C	Mildly active C
2.	35	2.7	2.2	CPH, fibrosis	CPH, lobular inflammation
3.	43	4.3	4.2	CAH, moderate severity	CPH
4.	49	6.3	6.3	CAH	Within normal limits
5.	43	.25	.25	CAH/C	CAH/C
		2.8	2.8		CPH
6.	32	.40	.40	Mild CAH	CAH, severe fibrosis
		4.4	4.4		NSR, fatty change
7.	51	.90	1.0	CAH (rule out C)	Mild CAH
		6.2	6.3		Mild portal/lob. inflam.
8.	35	.90	.80	Mild CAH	CPH
		6.4	6.3		CPH

CAH = chronic active hepatitis.
C = cirrhosis.
CPH = chronic persistent hepatitis.
NSR = non-specific reaction.

antiviral therapy. Polymerase chain reaction (PCR) has been used to detect persistent HBV DNA in liver, serum, or peripheral mononuclear cells because it is capable of amplifying specific DNA sequences and detecting small amounts of DNA which cannot be detected by direct hybridization.

Marcellin and associates looked for HBV DNA in serum, peripheral mononuclear cells, and liver of two patients who cleared HBsAg and HBV DNA (by dot blot hybridization) in response to treatment with adenine arabinoside monophosphate [6]. The authors found HBV DNA sequences in the serum and liver tissue 2 and 6 months after seroconversion. In a second study by the same investigators, HBV DNA was found in serum in 83 % of patients 6 or 12 months after loss of HBeAg but in only 15 % of patients 12 months after the disappearance of HBsAg [12]. In the Korenman study [7], 2 of 13 patients who became HBsAg negative as a result of interferon treatment were found to be PCR reactive in serum. Both of the HBV DNA positive patients underwent HBsAg to anti-HBs seroconversion within the previous 6 months whereas in the HBV DNA negative patients HBsAg loss had occurred 1 to 4 years earlier. Taken together, the above studies indicate that HBV DNA generally disappears from serum within one year after the disappearance of HBsAg.

Kuhns and associates established the long-term persistence of HBV DNA in liver tissue by using PCR to examine total hepatic DNA at remote intervals (2 to 6 years) after the disappearance of HBsAg [8]. The investigators found HBV DNA sequences in all but one of their patients. The Kuhns study was unique in that the authors used a modification of the solution hybridization assay to quantify the PCR product and found substantially lower levels of HBV DNA in liver tissue when compared to patients studied during the replicative phase of infection and a tendency for viral DNA levels to decrease with time. Mason and associates were able to detect HBV DNA by PCR in the peripheral mononuclear cells of several of the same patients, including two in which HBsAg disappeared 2 and 4 years earlier [13]. It is important to note that persistent HBV DNA was either detected in the peripheral blood mononuclear cells, liver, or both, of the cases collectively studied by Kuhns and Mason. More recently, Mason was able to detect viral mRNA in the liver of one of these patients 6 years after HBsAg clearance. The patient in question had detectable HBV DNA in serum as well, suggesting that on rare occasions low level viral replication may continue indefinitely [18].

Thus, after clearance of serum HBsAg, HBV DNA usually disappears in the serum, as detected by PCR, but it generally persists in liver tissue and occasionally also in peripheral mononuclear cells for prolonged intervals (Table II). Rarely, evidence for viral transcription may be detected in the liver years after clearance of serum HBsAg. The molecular state of the persistent HBV DNA, whether integrated into the host genome, in a closed circular state, or both has yet to be delineated. This has implications for viral reactivation and potential infectivity of these patients. The available studies have provided valuable insights into viral latency following loss of HBsAg from interferon therapy, but additional clinical and virological assessments are required to address the ultimate outcome of these patients.

*

* *

In conclusion, this paper describes the long-term clinical and virological outcomes in patients with chronic hepatitis B who respond to interferon therapy. Individuals who remain HBeAg positive but HBV DNA negative often undergo delayed clearance of HBeAg. Biochemical and virological remissions are generally maintained indefinitely in immunocompetent patients. Moreover, the frequency of HBsAg to anti-HBs seroconversion increases as the follow-up lengthens in responders. The degree

Table II. Immediate versus delayed effects in responders to interferon therapy.

Effect monitored	Short-term (≤ 12 mo after therapy)	Long-term
ALT/AST	Improved or within normal limits (1,2)	Improved or within normal limits (1,2)
Symptoms	Absent or improved (3,14)	Absent (3,14)
Histology	Diminished periportal necrosis (1,5)	Absent periportal necrosis (9, 10)
	Diminished portal reaction (1,5)	Slight or no portal reaction (9,10)
	Similar degree of fibrosis (1,5)	Diminished fibrosis (9,10)
HBeAg	Remains negative (1,2)	Remains negative (7,11)
		Delayed clearance in HBV DNA negative patients (3,11)
HBsAg	Clearance in minority (1,2)	Clearance common (3,7)
HBV nucleic acid by PCR		
Serum HBV DNA	Positive/negative (6,7,12)	Usually negative (7,8)
Liver tissue		
HBV DNA	Positive (6,8)	Usually positive (8,10)
HBV RNA	Positive/negative (18)	Usually negative (18)
PBMC†HBV DNA	Positive/negative (6,13)	Positive/negative (13)

† Peripheral blood mononuclear cells

of histological improvement years after a response is achieved is generally much greater than that found in short-term histological assessments. Using PCR, serum HBV DNA generally disappears at the time of or within a year after the disappearance of HBsAg. Small amounts of latent HBV DNA generally persist in liver tissue, however, and viral DNA sequences may occasionally be detected in circulating mononuclear cells years after the disappearance of HBsAg. At the current time it is not known whether latent HBV will have any future clinical consequences. Continued observation and further virological study are necessary to address this important question.

References

1. Hoofnagle JH, Peters M, Mullen KD, *et al.* Randomized, controlled trial of recombinant human alpha-interferon in patients with chronic hepatitis B. Gastroenterology 1988 ; 95 : 1318-25.
2. Perrillo RP, Schiff ER, Davis GL, *et al.* A randomized, controlled trial of interferon alfa-2b alone and after prednisone withdrawal for the treatment of chronic hepatitis B. N Engl J Med 1990 ; 323 : 295-301.
3. Perrillo RP. Antiviral agents in the treatment of chronic viral hepatitis. In : Boyer J, Ockner R, eds. Progress in liver diseases. New York : WB Saunders. Volume X, 1992 : 283-309.
4. Kuhns M, McNamara A, Cabal C, *et al.*A new assay for the quantitative detection of hepatitis B viral DNA in human serum. In : Zuckerman AJ, ed. Viral hepatitis and liver disease. New York : AR Liss, 1988 : 258-62.
5. Brook MG, Petrovic L, McDonald JA, Scheuer PJ, Thomas HC. Histological improvement after anti-viral treatment for chronic hepatitis B virus infection. J Hepatol 1989 ; 8 : 218-25.
6. Marcellin P, Martinot-Peignoux M, Loriot MA, *et al.* Persistence of hepatitis B virus DNA demonstrated by polymerase chain reaction in serum and liver after loss of HBsAg induced by antiviral therapy. Ann Intern Med 1990 ; 112 : 227-8.
7. Korenman J, Baker B, Waggoner J, Everhart JE, Di Bisceglie AM, Hoofnagle JH. Long-term remission of chronic hepatitis B after alpha-interferon therapy. Ann Intern Med 1991 ; 114 : 629-34.
8. Kuhns M, McNamara A, Mason A, Campbell C, Perrillo R. Serum and liver hepatitis B virus DNA in chronic hepatitis B after sustained loss of surface antigen. Gastroenterology 1992 ; 103 : 1649-56.
9. Perrillo RP, Brunt EM. Hepatic histologic and immunohistochemical changes in chronic hepatitis B after prolonged clearance of hepatitis B e antigen and hepatitis B surface antigen. Ann Intern Med 1991 ; 115 : 113-5.
10. Fong TL, Di Bisceglie AM, Feinstone SM, Axiotis CA, Hoofnagle JH. Persistent hepatic HBV-DNA after clearance of HBsAg from serum of patients with chronic hepatitis B. Hepatology 1991 ; 14 : 130 A (abstract).
11. Lok ASF, Chung HT, Liu VWS, Ma OCK. Long-term follow-up of chronic hepatitis B patients treated with alpha-interferon. Gastroenterology, in press.
12. Lorit MA, Marcellin P, Bismuth E, *et al.* Demonstration of hepatitis B virus DNA by polymerase chain reaction in the serum and liver after spontaneous or therapeutically induced HBeAg to anti-HBe or HBsAg to anti-HBs seroconversion in patients with chronic hepatitis B. Hepatology 1992 ; 15 : 32-6.
13. Mason A, Yoffee B, Noonan C, *et al.* Hepatitis B virus DNA in peripheral blood mononuclear cells in chronic hepatitis B after HBsAg clearance. Hepatology 1992 ; 16 : 36-41.
14. Perrillo RP. Antiviral therapy of chronic hepatitis B : past, present, and future. J Hepatol, in press.
15. Krogsgaard K, Lindhardt BO, Nielsen JO, *et al.* The influence of HTLV-III infection on the natural history of hepatitis B virus infection in male homosexual HBsAg carriers. Hepatology 1987 ; 7 : 37-41.
16. Brunetto MR, Oliveri F, Rocca G, *et al.* Natural course and response to interferon of chronic hepatitis B accompanied by antibody to hepatitis B e antigen. Hepatology 1989 ; 10 : 198-202.
17. Hadziyannis S, Bramou T, Makris A, Moussooulis G, Zigneno L, Papaioannou C. Interferon alfa-2b treatment of HBeAg negative/serum HBV DNA positive chronic active hepatitis type B. J Hepatol 1990 ; 11 : S133-6.
18. Mason A, Campbell C, Perrillo RP. Continued transcription of hepatitis B virus in the liver after clearance of serum HBsAg. Hepatology 1992 ; 16 : 127 A (abstract).

References

1. Hoofnagle JH, Peters M, Mullen KD, et al. Randomized, controlled trial of recombinant human alpha-interferon in patients with chronic hepatitis B. Gastroenterology 1988; 95: 1318-25.
2. Perrillo RP, Schiff ER, Davis GL et al. A randomized, controlled trial of interferon alfa-2b alone and after prednisone withdrawal for the treatment of chronic hepatitis B. N Engl J Med 1990; 323: 295-301.
3. [illegible]

Progress in Hepatology 93. J.P. Miguet and D. Dhumeaux, eds.
John Libbey Eurotext, Paris © 1993, pp. 55-61

6

Management of anti-HBe positive chronic hepatitis

F. BONINO, M.R.BRUNETTO

Department of Gastroenterology, Molinette Hospital, 10126 Torino, Italy.

Chronic anti-HBe positive hepatitis B was originally identified in 1981 when detection of HBV-DNA by molecular hybridization techniques was first introduced in clinical specimens [1]. Then it was defined as a specific clinical entity characterized by chronic hepatitis associated with intrahepatic HBcAg (frequently intracytoplasmic), HBV-DNA and IgM anti-HBc in serum [2]. The virological cause of the disease was finally identified in the chronic infection with HBeAg defective HBV mutants having a unique G-A switch at nucleotide 1896 of the pre-C region of the C gene of HBV-DNA [3, 4]. This mutation represents the major cause (> 95 %) of the lack of secretion of HBeAg in patients with chronic anti-HBe positive hepatitis B [5, 6]. The pathogenesis of anti-HBe chronic hepatitis does not differ from that of HBeAg positive form. The presence of HBeAg and anti-HBe in the serum of patients with chronic hepatitis B identifies two specific phases of the natural course of chronic HBV infection. Patients with one or the other form of liver disease have different rates of spontaneous and interferon induced recoveries [3, 5-6].

Diagnosis

The most important problem in the management of chronic hepatitis associated with serum anti-HBe is the etiologic diagnosis of liver disease. In fact anti-HBe can be associated with any form of liver disease even if the antibody is more frequently the hallmark of chronic hepatitis B caused by HBeAg defective HBV. The most reliable method to make a specific etiologic diagnosis of viral hepatitis would be to identify specific intrahepatic cytotoxic T lymphocytes responsible for the killing of virus infected hepatocytes. Unfortunately this cannot be proposed for routine diagnosis. Therefore we have to rely on surrogate tests. Detection of HBV and even of a consistent number of viruses does not imply necessarily that the liver damage is caused by HBV. In fact it is well known that florid HBV replication can persist for years without liver damage if the host's immune system does not react against virus antigens. This phase of HBV infection is usually called « immunotolerance ». Some patients may be HBV carrier in the immunotolerance phase but they can have other causes of liver damage. Therefore the hepatologist has to rely on specific markers of virus induced liver damage rather than on markers of virus infection and replication only. Since liver disease begins as soon as the immunotolerance is lost and virus infected cells begin to be eliminated (immunoelimination phase), for a highly specific etiologic diagnosis we have to use indirect markers of the host's antiviral immunoresponse, implicated in the virus induced liver damage. In both acute or chronic hepatitis patients, IgM antibodies against virus antigens implicated in virus immunoelimination appear suitable diagnostic tests. The improved sensitivity of new IgM anti-HBc tests allows the detection of this antibody with absolute sensitivity (10 UI, PEI) and IgM anti-HBc are found in any form of liver disease caused by HBV independently from the duration of virus infection and replication [7-12]. Elevated serum anti-HBc IgM levels (higher than 600 UI) are usually detected after acute flare-ups of alanine aminotransferases (2 to 4 weeks) that occur in primary hepatitis B and also in acutely relapsing chronic hepatitis B. This allows the identification of patients with either acute or chronic HBV induced liver disease, distinguishing them from HBsAg carriers with liver damage unrelated to HBV. All sera from HBsAg negative controls and HBsAg carriers without liver disease or patients with chronic hepatitis D have lower than 10 UI of IgM anti-HBc. Viremia and serum ALT and IgM anti-HBc levels fluctuate with significant peaks in patients with chronic anti-HBe positive hepatitis B and most of these patients have asymptomatic hepatitis B exacerbations that can be intervened by periods of uneventful disease with normal serum ALT levels. All episodes of ALT flare-ups are associated with an elevation of IgM anti-HBc levels (using quantitative automated assays sensitive enough to measure as low as 10 UI, PEI, of this antibody). The chronological sequence of events namely, HBV-DNA reactivation → ALT flare-up →IgM anti-HBc level increase warrants a specific etiologic diagnosis of hepatitis B exacerbations [11, 12]. This pattern helps to distinguish « true » hepatitis B exacerbations from ALT flare-ups or hepatitis episodes unrelated to HBV infection.

In fact no time relations are found among HBV-DNA, ALT and IgM anti-HBc fluctuations in chronic anti-HBe positive HBsAg carriers where hepatitis is caused by other viruses, HCV or HDV. In Table I, we summarize the specific tests that are used to make the etiologic diagnosis of chronic hepatitis B, C and D in anti-HBe positive patients.

Pathogenesis

Hepatitis B virus structural proteins are highly immunogenic and hepatitis B core antigen (HBcAg) is approximately 100-folds more immunogenic than HBsAg at both the T cell and B cell levels [8]. HBcAg is cross-reactive at the T cell level with its non-particulate secretory form, hepatitis B e antigen (HBeAg) [13]. HBV induces immunotolerance by overproduction of both envelope and nucleocapsid proteins. HBeAg/HBcAg-specific T cell tolerance is mediated by secretion of HBeAg that gains access to the thymus and can lead to the functional deletion of HLA class II-restricted, HBeAg/HBcAg-specific T helper cells (Th). This mechanism can explain the high rate of chronic HBV infection in newborns and the frequent loss of tolerance in young adults, chronic HBV carriers when a regressing thymus is no longer able to delete HBeAg/HBcAg-specific T cells. In the murine model, the degree of HBeAg/HBcAg-specific T cell tolerance is variable depending on the major histocompatibility complex (MHC) of the host.

These findings suggest that genetic variability of the immune system contributes to the different rates of spontaneous HBeAg to anti-HBe seroconversion in chronic HBV carriers. In longitudinal studies of chronic HBeAg positive carriers, HBeAg defective HBV appearance is frequently associated with the loss of immunotolerance and precedes the typical hepatitis B flare-up that leads to anti-HBe seroconversion [5,6].

Table I. Etiologic diagnosis of viral hepatitis (acute or chronic).

Serological markers of	HBV	HCV	HDV
Infection	HBsAg	anti-HCV	anti-HD
Replication	HBV-DNA	HCV-RNA	HDV-RNA
Disease	IgM anti-HBc	IgM anti-C22	IgM anti-HD

These observations prompted us to hypothesize that HBV mutants unable to secrete HBeAg represent one important cause of the loss of HBV immunotolerance. This hypothesis has been confirmed by recent studies of perinatal transmission of hepDNA virus infection in women and woodchucks. Newborns (to anti-HBe positive mothers) infected with mutant HBV (with stop codon at nucleotide 1896 of the pre-C region of HBV-DNA) developed self limited infections, while newborns (to HBeAg positive mothers) with wild-type HBV became chronic HBsAg carriers [14]. Newborn woodchucks infected with wild-type or mutant (the same stop codon as above) woodchuck hepatitis virus (WHV) developed respectively chronic (in 70 % of cases) or self limited infections (in all) (R. Miller *et al.*, NIH Bethesda, USA, personal communication).

All these data taken together suggest that HBV immunotolerance and chronic infection depend not only on the status and competence of the immune system, but also on HBV genetic heterogeneity (at least at nucleotide 1896 of the pre-C region of HBV-DNA). In fact fulminant hepatitis B has been described to occur in newborns to anti-HBe positive mothers infected with mixed virus populations containing relevant amounts of HBeAg defective virus [14].

In conclusion, HBeAg defective HBV appears to influence the outcome of primary HBV infection ; it is less likely than wild-type HBV to result in persistent infection but more likely to cause the virus immunoelimination and therefore liver injury. When virus tolerance is lost, the immunoelimination phase begins and infected hepatocytes are destroyed by HLA class I-restricted cytotoxic T lymphocyte (CTL) response to endogenously synthesized virus proteins (immunoelimination). T helper (Th) and CTL responses to HBcAg/HBeAg appear to play a major role in the HBV clearance and therefore in liver injury. During the immunoelimination phase the expression of HBeAg on the liver cell membrane of wild-type infected cells becomes a factor of negative selection. HBeAg defective variants as well as HBsAg variants are selected for under the pressure of the immune system. As the inflammatory reaction and disease progress, the relative proportions of HBeAg positive and negative viruses change so that mutant HBV becomes dominant. Eventually hepatocytes containing only HBeAg defective HBV will appear and escape immunoelimination, because they do not display a major target antigen of CTL response, HBeAg. This event entails the persistence of active HBV replication and liver damage in anti-HBe positive HBsAg carriers. In these patients, significant increases or reappearances of wild-type HBV are associated with hepatitis B exacerbations. In fact, in longitudinal studies, wild-type HBV was found to increase significantly before or at the time of the aminotransferase flare-ups while mutant HBV was selected for by the hepatitis B exacerbations. The positive selection of HBeAg defective HBV by the antiviral immunoreaction explains why a virus mutant, apparently deleterious for the persistence of chronic infection, is selected for in long lasting carriers of HBsAg.

Thus, many factors are implicated in each phase of hepatitis B pathogenesis and the duration of the phases varies from days to years. HBeAg defective HBV appears to be involved in the loss of virus tolerance and therefore in the pathogenesis of acute hepatitis B. In addition HBeAg defective is positively selected by both natural and interferon induced antiviral immunoreactions and behaving as an escape mutant it contributes also to the pathogenesis of severe chronic hepatitis B. The combination of all these characteristics explains the relative prevalence of this mutant over wild-type HBV in patients with severe acute hepatitis B and in chronic HBsAg carriers at the time of anti-HBe seroconversion and/or hepatitis B exacerbations. At the same time the absence of HBeAg defective mutants in some cases of severe and fulminant hepatitis B as well as its detection in asymptomatic carriers of HBsAg are not surprising. Chronic anti-HBe positive hepatitis B is specifically defined by detection of HBV replication markers and HBV induced liver damage in absence of HBeAg and it is in the great majority of cases caused by the ongoing infection with a prevalent HBV population of HBeAg defective viruses. The progressive selection of HBeAg defective virus prompted by a continuous but inefficacious antiviral immune reaction leads to the relative prevalence of the defective virus over wild-type HBV and lets HBV resist immunoelimination even more efficiently and perpetuate liver disease (Figure 1).

Therapy

The results of interferon treatment of 90 patients with chronic anti-HBe positive hepatitis included in four randomized controlled trials indicate that interferon inhibited HBV replication and ALT normalized in about 70 % of patients [15]. However, the effect of therapy was transient in the great majority of cases and hepatitis relapsed in 90 % of them. The analysis of factors predictive of response appears to confirm what has been observed in patients who have the HBeAg positive form of chronic hepatitis B. The worst type of response is associated with long lasting disease, cirrhosis and a relative prevalence of HBeAg defective virus

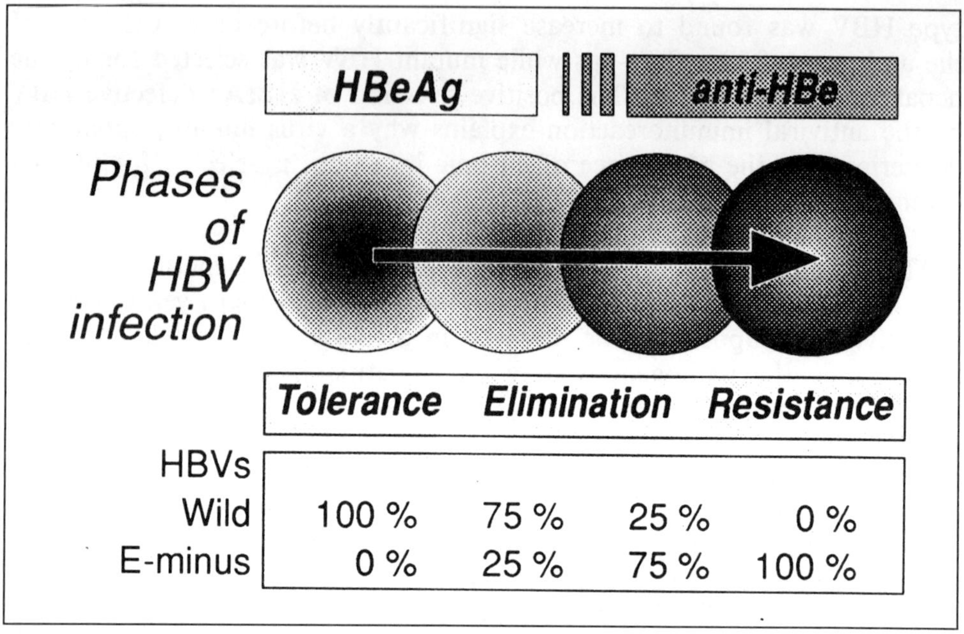

Figure 1. Successive phases of hepatitis B virus infection, from tolerance (wild-type virus) to immunoelimination resistance (HBeAg defective virus).

over wild-type in the infecting HBV population. The fact that resistance to virus elimination, duration of HBV-induced liver disease and severity of liver damage are all variables that depend on the prevalent infection of HBeAg defective HBV supports the view that such HBV mutant can be considered an interferon resistant virus. Therefore, genetic heterogeneity as for many other viruses represents for HBV one important factor of lack of response to therapy. This entails that interferon therapy should be started as soon as possible in the natural history of HBV infection at the time when the immunoelimination phase starts and before therapy resistant mutants are selected. Once therapy resistant HBV mutants become the prevalent virus population as in anti-HBe positive chronic hepatitis B, different therapeutic strategies including higher dose, longer duration and combinations of drugs have to be considered [15]. The results of ongoing clinical trials using new therapeutic schemes should provide more information in the near future.

References

Bonino F, Hoyer B, Nelson J, *et al.* Hepatitis B virus DNA in the sera of HBsAg carriers, a marker of active hepatitis B virus replication in the liver. Hepatology 1981 ; 1:386-91.

2. Bonino F, Rosina F, Rizzetto M, *et al.* Chronic hepatitis in HBsAg carriers with serum HBV-DNA and anti-HBe. Gastroenterology 1986 ; 90 :1268-73.
3. Brunetto MR, Stemler M, Schodel F, Will H, Ottobrelli A, Rizzetto M, Verme G, Bonino F. Identification of HBV variants which cannot produce precore derived HBeAg and may be responsible for severe hepatitis. Ital J Gastroenterol 1989 ; 21 : 151-4
4. Carman WF, Jacyna MR, Hadziyannis S, Karayannis P, McGarvey MJ, Makris A, Thomas J. Mutation preventing formation of hepatitis B e antigen in patients with chronic hepatitis B infection. Lancet 1989 ; 2 : 588-90.
5. Bonino FA, Brunetto MR, Purcell RH, Zuckerman AJ. Genetic heterogeneity of hepatitis viruses : clinical implications. J Hepatol Suppl.4 1991 ; 13 ; S1-174.
6. Brunetto MR, Giarin M, Oliveri F, Saracco G, Barbera C, Parrella T, Abate ML, Chiaberge E, Calvo PL, Manzini P, Verme G, Bonino F. « e » antigen defective hepatitis B virus and course of chronic infection. J Hepatol 1991 ; 13 (suppl 4) : S82-6.
7. Gerlich GH, Uy A, Lambrecht F, Thomssen R. Cut-off levels of IgM antibody against viral core antigen for differentiation of acute, chronic and past hepatitis B virus infections. J Clin Microbiol 1986 ; 24 : 288-93.
8. Tassopoulos NC, Sjogren MH, Ticehurst JR, Engle RE, Karayannis AR, Gerin JL, Purcell RH, Papaevangelou G. Significance of IgM antibody to hepatitis B core antigen in a Greek population with chronic hepatitis B virus infection. Liver 1986 ; 6 : 275-80.
9. Brunetto MR, Arrigoni A, Toti M, Almi P, Zanetti A, Ferroni P, Doris R, *et al.* The diagnostic significance of IgM antibody to hepatitis B core antigen, revisited. Ital J Gastroenterol 1986 ; 20 : 167.
10. Koike K, Lino K, Kurai K, Mitamura K, Endo Y, Oka H. IgM anti-HBc in anti-HBe positive chronic type B hepatitis with acute exacerbations. Hepatology 1987 ; 7 : 573-6.
11. Brunetto MR, Torrani Cerentia M, Olivieri F, Piantino P, Randone A, Calvo PL, *et al.* Monitoring the natural course and response to therapy of chronic hepatitis B with an automated semi-quantitative assay for IgM anti-HBc. J Hepatol 1993 ; in press.
12. Colloredo Mels G, Bellati G, Leandro G, Brunetto MR, Vicari O, Borzio M, Piantino P, Fornaciari G, Scudeller G, Angeli G, Bonino F, Ideo G. Kinetics of HBV-DNA, ALT and IgM anti-HBc during chronic hepatitis B reactivations. Submitted.
13. Bertoletti A, Ferrari C, Fiaccadori F, Penna A, Margolskee R, Schlicht HJ, Fowler P, Guilhot S, Chisari FV. HLA class I-restricted human cytotoxic cells recognize endogenously synthesized hepatitis B virus nucleocapsid antigen. Proc Natl Acad Sci USA 1991 ; 88 : 10445-9.
14. Raimondo G, Tanzi E, Brancatelli S, Campo S, Sardo MA, Rodino G, Pernice M, Zanetti AR. Is the course of perinatal hepatitis B virus infection influenced by genetic heterogeneity of the virus ? J Med Virol 1993 ; in press.
15. Brunetto MR, Oliveri F, Demartini A, Calvo PL, Manzini P, Torrani CM, Bonino F. Treatment with interferon of chronic hepatitis B associated with antibody to hepatitis B e antigen. J Hepatol Suppl. 1 1991 ; 13 : S8-11.

Progress in Hepatology 93. J.P. Miguet and D. Dhumeaux, eds.
John Libbey Eurotext, Paris © 1993, pp. 63-68

7

Pathophysiology of chronic hepatitis C

J. CAMPS, J. CÓRDOBA, J.I. ESTEBAN

Liver Unit, Hospital Vall d'Hebron, 08035 Barcelona, Spain.

In the absence of an *in vitro* cell culture system, the life cycle of the hepatitis C virus (HCV) at the cellular level remains largely unknown. However, despite our currently lack of knowledge of the interactions between HCV and the hepatocyte, a large amount of clinical, histological, biochemical, serological and immunological information (albeit fragmentary and sometimes conflicting) has accumulated through the study of natural infections (transfusion-associated or sporadic) in humans and, especially, through experimental infections in the chimpanzee (for review see references 1 and 2). Interpretation of this information, according to what we currently know about the nature of the HCV genome [3], may allow a reasonable attempt to address two basic aspects of this issue : the pathogenesis of HCV-induced liver damage and the possible mechanisms involved in viral persistence.

Mechanism(s) of liver cell injury

Whether HCV is directly cytopathic or whether the HCV-associated liver cell damage is immunologically mediated is still a matter of controversy.

Several observations strongly suggest that HCV replication may directly damage hepatocytes, without being necessarily cytolytic (enveloped viruses do not require lysing the host cell to release progeny virions). First, the general histological picture of chronic hepatitis C with predominant lobular inflammation, spotty, rather than bridging necrosis, frequent acidophilic bodies with minimal or no accompanying lymphocytic infiltrate along with scarce focal and patchy periportal piecemeal necrosis, is more suggestive of a cytopathic viral infection. This concept would be supported by the recent observation [4] in experimentally inoculated chimpanzees that detection of « replicating » HCV RNA by *in situ* hybridization coincides and parallels aminotransferase elevation, although it occurs in hepatocytes in the absence of morphological changes or inflammatory infiltrate during several weeks after inoculation, thus suggesting that HCV replication may somehow functionally damage hepatocytes (perhaps reversibly) without killing them. Third, the close correlation between biochemical response to alpha-interferon and concomitant loss of HCV RNA, the more severe course of HCV infection in immunocompromised individuals, and the demonstration in the chimpanzee model that changes in aminotransferase and HCV RNA levels in serum closely reflect HCV replication within the liver, all argue for a direct cytopathic effect. The frequent observation of persistent detection of HCV in serum, both in humans and chimpanzees, with normal aminotransferase levels and minimal unspecific changes or even normal liver histology, does not necessarily contradict direct cytopathicity. As discussed below, the emergence of mutants with a non-cytopathic phenotype might explain persistent low level replication of HCV in the absence of markers of liver cell damage.

On the other hand, there is ample evidence that HCV infection elicits a broad and strong humoral and cellular immune response to many HCV-encoded antigens, both in structural and non-structural viral proteins. Recent studies [5] have shown that in the majority of HCV-infected individuals, peripheral blood mononuclear cells exhibit a $CD4^+$ T cell proliferative response to several HCV-specific proteins, especially those encoded by the NS3 and NS4 regions, and a positive correlation has been observed between $CD4^+$ T cell response to core proteins and an apparently healthy carrier state (PCR-positive HCV carriers with persistently normal aminotransferase levels and normal liver histology). The presence of $CD8^+$ T cells with specific cytotoxic activity to several epitopes encoded by the E1, E2/NS1 and NS2 regions has been clearly demonstrated by directly cloning infiltrating lymphocytes from liver biopsy specimens of infected subjects [6]. This HCV-specific cytotoxic T lymphocytes (CTL), presumably present in high numbers within the infected liver, are capable of lysing allogenic lymphocytes infected with vaccinia virus constructs carrying HCV-peptides in a HLA-I restricted manner. Similarly, specific cytotoxic T cell responses to peptides encoded by the NS5 region of HCV has also been induced in a murine model immunized with a recombinant vaccinia-HCV-NS5 vector [7].

Hence, there seems to be no doubt that there is a host immune response against HCV infected cells which should be capable of recognizing and eliminating liver cells expressing a wide array of HCV-specific antigens. It is very likely that this immune response plays a significant role in protecting the infected liver from extensive HCV-induced damage, although in most cases it is unable to clear the infection. Despite its presumed ability to control HCV replication (to a certain level), the host immune response does not seem to protect the host from further reactivation of viral replication or from reinfection. This has been clearly shown in the chimpanzee model in several studies [8, 9]. Animals convalescent from an experimental HCV infection, who had normalized their enzyme activity and become serum HCV RNA negative, consistently develop evidence of active HCV infection (with returning viremia, histological changes and increase in antibody production) upon rechallenge with homologous or heterologous inocula. Although such experimental evidence has not been obtained in humans, several observations of multiple distinct episodes of acute non-A, non-B hepatitis have been described in drug abusers and in transfusion recipients, suggesting that humans are also unable to mount a protective immune response after apparent recovery from an episode of HCV infection. Furthermore, in the face of a persistent infection, the host's immune response might contribute or even play a key role in the progressive liver damage associated with chronic HCV infection. The frequent finding of lymphoid follicles within the portal tracts in biopsy specimens from patients with chronic hepatitis C, the persistent activation of sinusoidal lining cells, and the strong correlation between production of immune-mediated fibrogenic cytokines (like TGF-beta1) and the histological activity index [10], all suggest that the immune response of the infected host may play a fundamental role in the smoldering process which may eventuate in cirrhosis.

Mechanism(s) of viral persistence

In order to persist, HCV (like any virus) must accomplish two conditions. First, it must regulate its lytic potential and, second, it must avoid elimination by the host's immune system.

Due to its high mutation rate, estimated from sequence analysis of isolates obtained in patients and chimpanzees, at different times during chronic infection [11, 12], HCV may use a variety of strategies to fulfill both requirements. The mutation rate and potential for rapid evolution explains why HCV (like most RNA viruses that replicate through an error-prone

RNA-polymerase lacking proofreading activity) circulates as a heterogeneous mixture of closely related genomes containing a master (most frequently represented) sequence and a large spectrum of mutants, a genomic distribution referred to as « quasispecies » [13]. This quasispecies model of mixed RNA virus populations has important biological implications which may explain viral persistence. First, the simultaneous presence of multiple viral genomes (and the high rate of generation of new variants) may allow selection of mutants that can modulate the lytic potential of the « wild type virus » (which initiates and causes the acute hepatitis phase). An attractive example of this type of mutants is known as defective interfering particles (DIP). There are infectious particles, which are unable to replicate without the help of the wild type virus, because of deletions of genes essential for replication. Hence, DIP mutants coinfect cells and replicate at the expense of the helper virus, decreasing the viral yield, attenuating the cytopathic process and facilitating persistence. Although there is no experimental evidence for DIP of HCV during *in vivo* infection, the replication of HCV in infected individuals with normal enzyme activities and no evidence of overt ongoing liver damage strongly suggest that HCV quasispecies may generate non-cytopathic mutants.

Although there are several mechanisms by which viruses evade the immune system, the most likely strategy employed by HCV is the « antigenic drift », that is the continuous selection of neutralizing antibody and CTL escape mutants. This strategy would be in accordance with the extreme heterogeneity and rapid mutation rates observed in those genes coding for the two envelope glycoproteins, which would be the target epitopes for neutralization, antibody-dependent cell-mediated cytotoxicity and also specific $CD8^{+}$ T cell-mediated cytotoxicity of infected cells. One limitation to CTL escape is that epitopes for cell-mediated immunity may be present in any viral-encoded protein (not only envelope proteins) and the extent of mutation in regulatory proteins essential for viral replication is limited. However, as much as a single amino acid substitution within CTL epitopes has been shown to result in loss of recognition by virus-specific CTL, it is possible that sequence variation leads to escape from cellular immune recognition and contributes to viral persistence. Recent evidence [12] showing increasing complexity of the HCV quasispecies (i.e. accumulation of mutants with more divergent variation) in the hypervariable region of the envelope glycoprotein gp70, in sequential isolates of a chronically infected chimpanzee, strongly supports that antigenic drift is an important mechanism by which HCV escapes immune elimination.

Hence, sequence variation and quasispecies evolution may explain both attenuation and escape from immune elimination, and therefore viral persistence. It is likely that more than one mechanism underlies persistency. Several reports have suggested that HCV may infect peripheral blood mononuclear cells (PBMC), thus providing an additional strategy for viral persistence. However, in view of the complex predicted secondary structure of the 5' untranslated region of HCV and the potential for extensive base pairing, our lack of data concerning the steps unsolved in the replication of HCV, and the recent description of RNA heteroduplex formation in the 5' end of some single stranded RNA viruses, as an essential requirement for efficient encapsidation of the genome, the simple detection of minus-strand RNA segments in PBMC (which may contain genomic RNA during the process of removing virions or immune complexes from the circulation) does not prove tropism (and replication) of HCV in immune cells.

A hypothetical model of the pathophysiology of chronic hepatitis C

The two above mentioned mechanisms for hepatocellular damage and viral persistence could be integrated into a model in which a potentially cytopathic virus, with a high mutation rate capacity, generates a quasispecies (shortly after or during acute infection) which enables attenuation of the cytopathic phenotype, downregulation of replication, avoidance of immune elimination by the host and, hence, viral persistence. The subsequent course of events may be variable depending on the immune pressure exerted by the host, and possibly other factors (i.e. virus-cell coevolution). In young individuals and chronic infections of short-term duration, the infected host may be able to control viral replication to a level in which the viral quasispecies remains relatively stable for prolonged periods. During long-term infection, the continuous emergence of immune escape mutants would generate an even more complex quasispecies, perhaps with emergence of mutants reverting to more cytopathic phenotypes. In trying to keep replication under control, the host immune response may induce hepatocellular damage and stimulate release of fibrogenic cytokines which will induce production and deposition of collagen produced by fat-storing cells, fibroblasts, etc. At the same time, immunological abnormalities may develop, some of them having no clinicopathological significance (many types of autoantibodies), and some, including secondary immune processes of clinical relevance (cryoglobulinemia). Long-standing infections may eventuate in the establishment of liver cirrhosis, which in the absence of aggravating cofactors such as alcoholism, may evolve insidiously with preservation of liver function for many years.

It is also possible that during chronic infections, accumulation of defective interfering particles of replication of incompetent mutants leads to recovery or establishment of latent non-productive infection.

References

1. Esteban JI, Genescà J, Alter HJ. Hepatitis C : molecular biology, pathogenesis, epidemiology, clinical features, and prevention. In : Boyer JL, Ockner RK, eds. Progress in liver diseases. Vol. 10. Philadelphia : WB Saunders, 1992 : 253-82.
2. Bradley DW. Hepatitis non-A, non-B viruses become identified as hepatitis C and E viruses. In : Melnick JL, ed. Progress in medical virology. Vol. 37. Basel : Karger, 1990 : 101-35.
3. Houghton M, Weiner A, Han J, Kuo G, Choo QL. Molecular biology of the hepatitis C viruses : implications for diagnosis, development and control of viral disease. Hepatology 1991 ; 14 : 381-8.
4. Negro F, Pacchioni D, Shimizu Y, *et al.* Detection of intrahepatic replication of hepatitis C virus RNA by *in situ* hybridization and comparison with histopathology. Proc Natl Acad Sci USA 1992 ; 89 : 2247-51.
5. Botarelli P, Brunetto MR, Minutello MA, *et al.* T-lymphocyte response to hepatitis C virus in different clinical courses of infection. Gastroenterology 1993 ; 104 : 580-7.
6. Koziel MJ, Dudley D, Wong JT, *et al.* Intrahepatic cytotoxic T lymphocytes specific for hepatitis C virus in persons with chronic hepatitis. J Immunol 1992 ; 149 : 3339-44.
7. Shirai M, Akatsuka T, Pendleton CD, *et al.* Induction of cytotoxic T cells to a cross-reactive epitope in the hepatitis C virus nonstructural RNA polymerase-like protein. J Virol 1992 ; 66 : 4098-106.
8. Prince A, Brotman B, Huima T, Pascual D, Jaffery M, Inchauspe G. Immunity in hepatitis C infection. J Infect Dis 1992 ; 165 : 438-43.
9. Farci P, Alter HJ, Govindarajan S, *et al.* Lack of protective immunity against reinfection with hepatitis C virus. Science 1992 ; 258 : 135-40.
10. Castilla A, Prieto J, Fausto N. Transforming growth factors beta1 and alfa in chronic liver disease. N Engl J Med 1991 ; 324 : 933-40.
11. Ogata N, Alter HJ, Miller RH, Purcell RH. Nucleotide sequence and mutation rate of the H strain of hepatitis C virus. Proc Natl Acad Sci USA 1991 ; 88 : 3392-6.
12. Okamoto H, Kojima M, Okada SI, *et al.* Genetic drift of hepatitis C virus during an 8.2-year infection in a chimpanzee : variability and stability. Virology 1992 ; 190 : 894-9.
13. Martel M, Esteban JI, Quer J, *et al.* Hepatitis C virus circulates as a population of different but closely related genomes. Quasispecies nature of HCV genome distribution. J Virol 1992 ; 66 : 3225-9.

Progress in Hepatology 93, J.P. Miguet and D. Dhumeaux, eds.
John Libbey Eurotext, Paris © 1993, pp. 69-77

8

Factors of response to antiviral treatments in chronic hepatitis C

C. TREPO[1, 2], F. HABERSETZER[1], F. BAILLY[1], F. BERBY[2], C. PICHOUD[2], P. BERTHILLON[2], L. VITVITSKI[2]

[1] *Service d'Hépato-Gastroentérologie, Hôpital de l'Hôtel-Dieu, 69288 Lyon Cedex 2, France ;*
[2] *Unité de Recherche sur les Hépatites et les Rétrovirus Humains (INSERM U 271), 69424 Lyon Cedex 3, France.*

Definitions and relevance of end points

The natural history of chronic hepatitis C leads to progressive inflammation of the liver with development of cirrhosis and its complications including hepatocellular carcinoma [1]. There is an extreme variability in the proportion of cases with progressive liver disease and in the pace of that evolution. Most studies indicate that 20 % of chronic hepatitis C cases do develop liver cirrhosis. However, in a long-term follow-up study carried out by Seeff *et al.*, no significant mortality related to hepatitis C could be demonstrated over a 20-year period [2].

This calls for a careful definition of end points in all the trials devoted to the therapy of chronic hepatitis C. Ideally, the true end points of therapy should be to abolish the cause of the disease, i.e. eradicate HCV infection and suppress its consequences, liver necrosis and inflammation, fibrosis and cirrhosis. After many years, this outcome may be associated with different symptoms due to impairment of liver function as well as extrahepatic manifestations.

Reduction of morbidity and mortality is the objective of therapy. Such goals are most difficult to reach, and because of the long duration of the disease they cannot be chosen as end points of prospective studies since they would take several decades. Moreover, as suggested from the retrospective studies, they would lead to nonsignificant results and therefore will never be carried out.

All the studies published so far have used only readily available markers such as alanine aminotransferase (ALT) and histological scores, usually the Knodell score [3]. It should be emphazised that these have to be considered as convenient markers only.

Since true end points, i.e. morbidity and mortality, cannot be used, it is critically important to select which end points may be the most relevant as surrogate markers for therapeutical trials. As suggested before, we should select them by taking into consideration the suppression of both the cause and the consequences of the disease. The ultimate markers therefore should be those who can allow direct appraisal of viral replication in qualitative and quantitative terms, i.e. a quantitative estimation of HCV RNA in serum and liver for each of the genotypes.

As far as the consequences of viral infection in the liver are concerned, ALT may be both convenient and misleading since HCV is probably not directly cytopathic as indicated by many recent studies. Necrosis and inflammation of the liver are relevant parameters and the Knodell score is aiming at their quantification. Unfortunately, this score has many limits and flaws, especially in chronic hepatitis C. Cirrhosis is of critical importance but it is a very late marker and it is crippled, as all histological parameters, by the frequency of sampling errors in liver biopsies. Fibrosis is most crucial but it is most difficult to assess and it is certainly the least used of all histological parameters.

These conceptual considerations are of utmost importance for the interpretation of all the clinical trials which have been carried out so far. As we will see in the following definitions, these have mainly focused on ALT. Any extrapolation from this imperfect marker is therefore hazardous and potentially misleading.

Three types of responses to therapy are usually distinguished. A complete response is defined as normalization of ALT within a few weeks to 6 months of therapy. It is called sustained if it can be maintained for more than 6 months after cessation of treatment. Remarkably this definition usually neither takes into account elimination of HCV RNA nor the liver histological benefit. Partial response is usually defined as reduction of 50 % of base line ALT values. However, this is a loose definition since ALT are highly fluctuating and base lines are too often short and poorly defined. Some studies have considered as complete response cases in which ALT became normal at only one point in time. Another trend has also been to coin the term « near complete response » for cases with ALT less than 1.5 the upper limit of normal. Lack of response is the easiest group to characterize by persistency of ALT at similar level.

Relapses design patient which normalized ALT during therapy but returned to abnormal levels during follow-up, while breakthroughs refer to secondary rise of ALT during therapy.

Impact of interferon regimen and heterogeneity of response to interferon

The main factors which determine the response rate are certainly the modalities of interferon therapy. Initial open studies have been followed by controlled, randomized studies with or without placebo. If we pool these studies altogether using different regimen and different situations, the complete response rate varies from 23 % to 87 % with a relapse rate of 25 % to 75 % in such responders. A metaanalysis involving 916 patients, enrolled in 17 studies [4], indicated that around 50 % of patients respond to interferon recombinant alpha by normalizing ALT at the end of therapy. Half of these will relapse within the 6 months of follow-up after cessation of treatment. Histological improvement is present in over 60 % of complete responders with significant decrease of inflammation and necrosis [4, 5]. Quite remarkably, this histological improvement is not strictly correlated with the ALT response and in fact histological benefit has been proven to be almost identical in cases which normalized ALT and in those with near complete response. Although the many studies published provide very different results, both dose and duration of treatment are critical in the response to therapy.

Dose

Initial trials compared 1 MU or 3 MU thrice weekly for 6 months [6-9]. More recent studies in Japan [10] have showed that higher doses up to 10 MU may provide more effective response than those obtained with lower doses thrice weekly. The Japanese authors insist that, at the induction phase, the daily dosage followed later by thrice weekly schedule was superior to other therapy modalities. This however awaits further confirmation.

Although higher doses have been suggested to be more active, escalating doses have permitted to obtain about only a small proportion of additional complete responders [11].

Duration of therapy

It has also been proved to be important for achieving sustained response. The impact of duration of therapy requires a careful analysis. In fact, several authors have failed to see a beneficial response of 12 *versus* 6 months if they were pooling all the cases together [12, 13]. However, if patients without cirrhosis were singled out, a significant benefit was obtained in those treated for 12 *versus* 6 months. 43.2 % of complete durable responders *versus* 16.7 % in the cirrhotic group [14].

Whether an induction therapy and a maintenance regimen should be distinguished has been the topic of several studies. Higher initial doses may be followed by lower relapse rates. Although a 1 MU dose was suggested to be able to maintain normal ALT follow-up, this did not hold true. Recent studies do suggest that a maintenance dose of 3 MU is better than 1 MU between the 6 th and 12 th months [14, 15]. This is also consistent with the results of Carreno *et al.* and Piazza *et al.* [16, 17].

Titrating the maintenance dose on the ALT values turned out to be deceitful. This is not surprising and emphasizes once more that ALT is a poor surrogate marker for HCV replication. In the study by Poynard, it has been shown that a maintenance therapy at 3 MU was more efficacious than discontinuation and retreatment at 3 MU to obtain complete ALT normalization and sustained remissions [15].

Heterogeneity of responses in centers using identical protocols and recombinant interferon

In the early randomized studies, four groups in Europe and the USA used an identical protocol with alpha-2b. They obtained different results. While in two studies 3 MU were better than 1 MU [6, 7], this was not found in the other two [8, 9]. Response rates varied from 23 % to 50 % between Lyons and Paris for example. This emphasizes that the category of patients treated was certainly as important in the outcome as the therapy regimen itself and prompted the search for predictive factors.

Predictive factors for response to interferon

An intensive search for such factors was conducted by several groups. Initially, in our first controlled study, we had been able to demonstrate that cirrhosis was a crucial factor in response to therapy [7]. Although initially a source of controversy, that was further confirmed by all recent investigations. A multiple step logistic regression analysis was carried out between Lyons and Paris. Absence of cirrhosis, young age, female sex and presence of lobular hepatitis were all associated with better response to interferon.

The problem of sex remains a questionable issue since female had a lower mean body weight and this may be in part an indirect consequence of higher dosage. It can also (like for HBV) translate a genuine biological phenomenon.

Relation of age with severity of disease and cirrhosis deserves further attention

In two studies using multivariate analysis, young age and absence of cirrhosis were consistently found to predict long-term response to interferon [18, 19]. The similar finding on the impact of severity of liver disease is again reported by Iino *et al.* from Japan and from the USA by Davis *et al.* Whether age and progression of liver disease may be completely separated remains to be critically evaluated.

Duration of disease

This parameter is most difficult to assess since it is only known in post-transfusion situation, in this mostly asymptomatic condition. Very early therapy for acute HCV infection does suggest that response to interferon at this early stage is mostly beneficial [20-23].

As far as chronic hepatitis C is concerned, two studies may indicate that in fact duration of disease may be important. In an early report from Japan, this appears to be the case with response in patients treated within a mean duration of 3.5 years [10, 24]. Another therapy study, carried out in France, in which patients were treated within an average of 18 months after onset, has shown an amazing proportion of sustained remission 2 years after a one-year course of interferon at moderate dose.

The analysis of that trial indeed suggested that the most unique factor possibly accounting for this exceptional response rate could be the early therapy [25].

Virological factors

As indicated in the introduction, these must not be considered as surrogate marker but as potential true end point. They deserved therefore maximum attention. Levels of different anti-HCV antibodies have been found to decline somewhat with therapy but those changes appeared to be slow and could not be correlated with response by using ELISA test. When turning to quantification of Western blot based assays, a more significant trend could be observed, especially with C100 and C33 antibodies. Such trends should be however improved when correlated with more acurate markers than ALT normalization. It is remarkable that in the study of Omata *et al.* in acute infection [20] all patients who cleared HCV RNA subsequently cleared anti-NS4, NS3 antibodies. New tests including IgM anti-capsid antibodies or IgG anti-envelope or anti-NS5 proteins may turn out to be much more useful in the future [26].

Far more important is the impact of HCV genotype on the interferon response. Many studies have recently focused on this and they do suggest that genotype is of utmost importance in the response to interferon. Using the Okamamoto classification, which has been widely used so far, chronic hepatitis associated with genotype type II was found to be the most resistant to interferon. In our own study we did find a dramatic difference between the interferon responses to genotypes I and II, the most prevalent ones in France. That difference did remain significant after multiple variable analysis as well as age and severity of liver disease.

Japanese workers have found that genotype IV responded similarly to type I while type III was the most responsive genotype to interferon therapy [27-29].

The pretreatment level of HCV RNA, when carefully quantified, appears to be also correlated to interferon response, especially if replaced within the frame of a specific genotype. In a recent study [30], which reanalyzed sera from the early multicenter US trial [6], it appeared that patients with a sustained complete response to interferon alpha therapy had lower treatment viremia levels than complete responders who relapsed after the drug was stopped ($p < 0.001$) or non-responders. High viremia levels were not related to the histological diagnosis but were associated with specific features of HCV infection including lobular inflammation, lymphoid aggregates and bile ducts lesions [30].

Although titration of HCV RNA is the most important issue, a merely qualitative determination will be also useful. In most of the complete responders HCV RNA is cleared soon after ALT normalizes. It has been documented that in some patients, viremia can still be detected by PCR, although ALT may remain normal for some time. Prospective studies have however shown that a secondary increase in ALT is common in that situation. By contrast, less than 10 % of complete responders are prone to late reactivation of hepatitis if HCV RNA remains negative for 6 months after cessation of therapy. While negativation of HCV RNA in serum and in liver at the end of treatment is not predictive of sustained remission, it becomes so after 6 months.

Finally, demonstration of HCV antigen in the liver by immunostaining has been found positive in more than 80 % of liver biopsies from patients who have chronic hepatitis C. Pretreatment levels of HCV antigen appear to be lower in patients responsive to interferon therapy [31] and expression of HCV antigen decreases in the liver of patients responding to therapy. It is in the cases in which HCV antigen cannot be detected prior therapy that the best response and longest sustained remission were observed.

Responses to other interferons and antiviral agents

It has been suggested that differences in responses may exist between different types of interferons. So far, evidence for that remains scanty. It is known that natural human interferon is not a single entity and is composed of a family of proteins. Lymphoblastoid interferon-alpha may contain different molecules. Whether this could turn out to be important in the response is the subject of prospective comparative randomized studies. Whether the response to interferon-beta will be identical to alpha and whether some failures with interferon-alpha may be rescued by interferon-beta has been suggested in anecdotal cases but this remains to be further substantiated.

It has also been suggested that the emergence of neutraziling anti-interferon antibodies may account for some breakthroughs. On theoretical ground it is conceivable that multivalent interferon preparation may overcome some of the neutralizing effects of anti-alpha 2a or alpha 2b antibodies. The response to ribavirin may be completely different than the response to interferon. Indeed several investigators have noticed that patients not responding to interferon-alpha recombinant may well respond to ribavirin. Factors of predictive response to ribavirin remain to be substantiated.

References

1. Alter HJ, Purcell RH, Shih JW, *et al.* Detection of antibody to hepatitis C virus in prospectively followed transfusion recipients with acute and chronic non-A, non-B hepatitis. N Engl J Med 1989 ; 321 : 1494-500.
2. Seeff LB, Buskell-Bales Z, Wright EC, *et al.* Long-term mortality after transfusion-associated non-A, non-B hepatitis. N Engl J Med 1992 ; 327 : 1906-11.
3. Knodell RG, Ishak KG, Black WC, *et al.* Formulation and application of a numerical scoring system for assessing histological activity in asymptomatic chronic active hepatitis. Hepatology 1981 ; 1 : 431-5.
4. Tinè F, Magrin S, Craxi A, Pagliaro L. Interferon for non-A, non-B hepatitis. A meta-analysis of randomized clinical trials. J Hepatol 1991 ; 13 : 192-9.
5. Di Bisceglie AM, Mornese A, Michetti P, *et al.* Treatment of chronic NANB (type C) hepatitis with recombinant interferon-alpha-2b. Preliminary clinical results. Gastroenterology 1990 ; 98 : A581.
6. Davis GL, Balart LA, Schiff ER, *et al.* Treatment of chronic hepatitis C with recombinant interferon-alpha. A multicenter randomized controlled trial. N Engl J Med 1989 ; 321 : 1501-6.
7. Causse X, Godinot H, Chevallier M, *et al.* Comparison of 1 or 3 MU interferon alpha-2b and placebo in patients with chronic non-A, non-B hepatitis. Gastroenterology 1991 ; 101 : 497-502.
8. Marcellin P, Boyer N, Giostra E, *et al.* Recombinant human alpha-interferon in patients with chronic non-A, non-B hepatitis : a multicenter randomized controlled trial from France. Hepatology 1991 ; 13 : 393-7.
9. Sarraco G, Rosina F, Torrani Cerenzia MR, *et al.* A randomized controlled trial of interferon alpha 2b as therapy for chronic non-A, non-B hepatitis. J Hepatol 1990 ; 11 : S43-9.
10. Iino S, Hino K, Kuroki T, Suzuki H, Yamamoto S, Ogawa N. Treatment of chronic hepatitis C with high dose interferon-alph-2b : a multicenter study. Viral hepatitis management : standards for the future, Cannes, 22-23 mai 1992.
11. Brouwer JT, Kleter GEM, Elewaut A, *et al.* Initial non-response to interferon in chronic hepatitis C : induction of ALT normalization and HCV-RNA disappearance by high-dose interferon therapy. J Hepatol 1992 ; 16 : S49.
12. Métreau JM and the French Group for the Study of NANB/C Chronic Hepatitis Treatment. Viral hepatitis management : standards for the future, Cannes, 22-23 mai 1992.
13. Craxi A, Di Marco O, Lo Iacono O, *et al.* Lymphoblastoid alpha-interferon for post-transfusion chronic hepatitis C : a randomized trial of 6 vs 12 months treatment. J Hepatol 1992 ; 16 : S8.
14. Jouët P, Roudot-Thoraval F, Dhumeaux D, Métreau JM and the French Group for the Study of NANB/C Chronic Hepatitis Treatment. J Hepatol 1992 ; 16 : S50.
15. Poynard T (personal communication).
16. Carreno V, Trépo C, Gerken G, *et al.*. A double blind placebo-controlled multicenter trial of treatment of chronic hepatitis NANB with recombinant interferon alpha-2a (ROFERON-A). Hepatology 1992 ; 16 : 75A.
17. Piazza M, Tosone G, Tisco D, *et al.* Therapy of chronic hepatitis C with recombinant interferon alpha-2b. Viral hepatitis management : standards for the future, Cannes, 22-23 mai 1992.

18. Cammà C, Craxi A, Tinès F, *et al.* Predictors of response to alpha interferon (IFN) in chronic hepatitis C : a multivariate analysis on 361 treated patients. Hepatology 1992 ; 16 : 131A.
19. Degott C, Giostra E, Chevallier M, *et al.* Effets de l'interféron alpha sur les lésions histologiques de l'hépatite chronique C : recherche de lésions prédictives de la réponse au traitement. Gastroenterol Clin Biol 1991 ; 15 : 895.
20. Omata M, Yokosuta O, Takano S, *et al.*. Resolution of acute hepatitis C after therapy with natural beta interferon. Lancet 1991 ; 338 : 914-5.
21. Esteban R. Is there a role for interferon in acute disease ? Viral hepatitis management : standards for the future, Cannes, 22-23 mai 1992.
22. Colombo M. A multicenter randomized controlled trial of recombinant interferon alpha-2b in patients with acute post-transfusion NANB/C hepatitis. Viral hepatitis management : standards for the future, Cannes, 22-23 mai 1992.
23. Viladomiu L, Genesca J, Esteban JI, *et al.* Interferon-alpha in acute post-transfusion hepatitis C : a randomized controlled trial. Hepatology 1992 ; 15 : 767-9.
24. Iino S. Treatment of chronic hepatitis C with interferon. International Symposium on viral hepatitis and liver disease (the 8th Triennial Congress), Tokyo, May 10-14, 1993. Scientific Program and Abstract Volume, P 16 : 44.
25. Poynard T, Bedossa P, Mathurin P, *et al.* Efficacy of long-term recombinant interferon-alpha in patients with chronic hepatitis C. A clinical, biological, histological and immunohistological study. Gastroenterol Clin Biol 1991 ; 15 : 615-9.
26. Hellström UB, Sylvan SPE, Decker RH, *et al.* Immunoglobulin M reactivity towards the immunologically active region SP75 of the core protein of hepatitis C virus (HCV) in chronic HCV infections. J Med Virol 1993 ; 39 : 325-32.
27. Okamoto H, Sugiyama Y, Okada S, *et al.* Typing hepatitis C virus by polymerase chain reaction with type-specific primers : application to clinical surveys and tracing infectious sources. J Gen Virol 1992 ; 73 : 673-9.
28. Kanai K, Kako M, Okamoto H. HCV genotypes in chronic hepatitis C and response to interferon. Lancet 1992 ; 339 : 1543.
29. Yoshioka K, Kakumu S, Wakita T, *et al.* Detection of hepatitis C virus by polymerase chain reaction and response to interferon-α therapy : relationship to genotypes of hepatitis C virus. Hepatology 1992 ; 16 : 293-9.
30. Lau JYN, Davis GL, Kniffen J, *et al.* Significance of serum hepatitis C virus RNA levels in chronic hepatitis C. Lancet 1993 ; 341 : 1501-4.
31. Krawczynski K, Beach MJ, Bradley DW, *et al.* Hepatitis C virus antigen in hepatocytes : immunomorphologic detection and identification. Gastroenterology 1992 ; 103 : 622-9.

Progress in Hepatology 93. J.P. Miguet and D. Dhumeaux, eds.
John Libbey Eurotext, Paris © 1993, pp. 79-87

9

Autoimmunity and hepatitis C virus

M. P. MANNS

Department of Gastroenterology and Hepatology,
Zentrum Innere Medizin und Dermatologie, D-3000 Hannover 61, Germany.

Since the identification of the hepatitis C virus (HCV) in 1989, our knowledge concerning the molecular structure of this virus has increased tremendously. Among the most exciting areas is the interaction between HCV and the immune system. So far we know very little about the mechanisms that lead to tissue destruction by HCV infection, in particular to what extent the virus itself is cytopathic or to which extent immune reactions towards virus-infected cells contribute to liver cell damage. Of particular interest is the interaction between HCV and the immune system as well as the involvement of HCV in the induction of autoimmunity. Furthermore, HCV becomes involved in an increasing number of non-hepatic diseases, many of them are believed to have an autoimmune background. Among them are mixed cryoglobulinemia, porphyria cutanea tarda, Sjögren's syndrome and lately membranoproliferative glomerulonephritis. The list of such diseases is not complete, yet. Probably many others will follow. HCV shares many similarities with pestiviruses which in veterinary medicine are responsible for numerous deleterious diseases affecting different organ systems, in particular in the pig. The present article will review our knowledge on the link between HCV infection and autoimmunity in liver disease as well as the involvement of HCV in non-hepatic diseases of potential autoimmune background.

Hepatitis C virus in autoimmune liver diseases

In the early days of anti-HCV antibody testing by first generation ELISA assays, positive HCV results were obtained in all groups of autoimmune liver diseases [1]. The results were reported from different geographical areas. McFarlane and coworkers [2] first identified the frequent false positive anti-HCV results due to hypergammaglobulinemia. Later, when more specific and sensitive anti-HCV antibody testing became available and HCV-RNA testing by polymerase chain reaction assay was added to the diagnostic procedures, it became evident that the percentage of positivity depended on the geographical origin of the patients. HCV infection does not seem to play a major role in patients from Northern Europe and Northern America. In Southern Europe and in Japan where the prevalence of HCV infection is high, HCV markers are found in all groups of autoimmune liver diseases. However, the association of HCV infection became particularly relevant in autoimmune hepatitis type 2 which is associated with LKM-1 autoantibodies. LKM-1 autoantibodies are directed against a particular drug metabolizing enzyme, cytochrome P450 IID6. In Japan [3] and possibly in Africa (unpublished data), HCV infection may lead to the induction of antinuclear antibodies. It is unknown whether this is due to a particular HCV strain or to a particular genetic background.

Hepatitis C virus and autoimmune hepatitis type 2

When HCV-RNA determination is used as a confirmatory test, the only significant association of HCV infection with autoimmune liver disease is with LKM-1 antibody positive autoimmune hepatitis type 2. There is also a geographical difference. While HCV infection in autoimmune hepatitis type 2 is very low (< 10 %) in England [4], it is around 50 % in Germany [5] and France [6] while the association of autoimmune hepatitis type 2 with HCV infection is more than 90 % in Italy [4], Spain, and Japan [7]. In North America, the Caucasian population as investigated at the Mayo Clinic in Rochester exhibits a very low HCV association similar to England [8] while the situation in more Southern parts of the USA, i.e. Florida, reflects more the situation in Southern Europe.

Clinically HCV negative cases with autoimmune hepatitis type 2 resemble more the classical characteristics of autoimmune hepatitis, i.e. patients are young females, they respond to immunosuppression, disease activity is high, and prognosis is bad when patients are untreated. Extrahepatic clinical autoimmune syndromes are common [9, 10]. On the other hand, HCV positive cases with LKM-1 antibodies share many clinical characteristics of transfusion acquired HCV infection : milder disease, no profound female predominance and little if any response to immunosuppression. In addition LKM-1 antibody titers are much lower in HCV positive than in HCV negative cases [5]. This HCV positive group of patients with LKM-1 antibody positive autoimmune hepatitis was also called type 2 b [5]. The association of this subgroup with HCV infection was supported by the specific detection of anti-GOR in this autoimmune hepatitis type 2 b (see below).

Concerning immunogenetics, the situation is less clear. As early as 1987 when HCV testing was not available, Homberg and coworkers [9] described an increased incidence of HLA DR 3 in autoimmune hepatitis type 2. Last year we found a significant increase in HLA DR3 only in the HCV negative group while in both HCV positive and HCV negative cases C4A-Q0 alleles are increased [11]. In Italian patients HLA DR3 was also increased in the HCV positive cases with autoimmune hepatitis type 2 [12].

HCV associated autoimmune hepatitis type 2 and response to treatment

Several reports have documented the potential risk of LKM-1 positive liver disease to be deteriorated when treated with interferons. We have reported one child from Spain that deteriorated when treated with interferon because of hepatitis non A, non B [13]. Similar cases have been reported from several centers in Italy ([14], Bianchi *et al.* unpublished, Rizzetto *et al.*, unpublished). The general experience is that HCV positive cases with LKM-1 antibody positive autoimmune hepatitis type 2 do not profit from immunosuppression either with corticosteroids alone or in combination with azathioprine [5]. There is uncertainty on the efficacy of interferon treatment in these HCV-RNA and LKM-1 antibody positive cases. Usually interferons are well tolerated and normalization of transaminases may be observed. Usually these patients do not become long-term responders (Durazzo, Rizzetto *et al.* and Bianchi *et al.*, personal communication).

Specificity of microsomal autoantigens in HCV associated liver disease

LKM-1 autoantibodies were shown to react mainly with a 50 KD microsomal protein. This 50 KD major target antigen was identified as cytochrome P 450 IID6 [15, 16]. The major B cell epitope on cytochrome P 450 IID6 has a sequence of 8 aminoacids which shares extensive sequence homology with the immediate early protein of the herpes simplex virus type 1 [17]. This major B cell epitope is recognized by all HCV negative cases. HCV positive cases with autoimmune hepatitis type 2 have lower autoantibody titers as indicated above. Usually LKM-1 antibodies from HCV positive cases recognize a slightly larger sequence on cytochrome P 450 IID6, some of these sera did not recognize recombinant cytochrome P 450 IID6 at all [17]. Some authors have reported that LKM-1 antibodies in HCV positive liver disease do not react with P 450 IID6 [18]. Very recently we have shown that LKM-1 antibodies in HCV positive autoimmune hepatitis type 2 recognize 50 KD P 450 IID6, or additional proteins at 59 and 70 KD [19]. Some LKM-1 sera giving the typical fluorescence pattern on liver and kidney tissue do not react in Western blotting with any specific microsomal band. Possibly these microsomal autoantibodies recognize a conformational epitope. At present our laboratory is involved in cloning experiments for these additional microsomal antigens.

It is of particular interest whether these differences in the reactivity with microsomal antigens may correlate with the patient's response to interferon treatment. Preliminary data suggest that patients with reactivity towards the 50 and 70 KD antigens have a better response to immunosuppression [19]. These preliminary data have to be confirmed.

Is the anti-GOR response specific for hepatitis C virus infection ?

Mishiro *et al.* [20] prepared a cDNA library from a serum of a chimpanzee with chronic hepatitis C virus infection. The chimpanzee had been inoculated with serum from a blood donor who had transmitted hepatitis non A, non B to other patients. Screening this cDNA library with the serum from a patient with chronic hepatitis non A, non B resulted in a cDNA clone. The recombinant protein derived from this cDNA clone reacted with sera from patients with acute and chronic hepatitis C. Since this cDNA reacted with the non-infected chimpanzee's liver, it was concluded that GOR antigen is a self antigen. Since the anti-GOR response occurred in serum before the appearance of classical anti-HCV antibodies in acute hepatitis C, the authors discussed whether anti-GOR could be used in the diagnosis of acute hepatitis C and when screening blood donors.

The specificity of the anti-GOR response for HCV virus infection is supported by several observations. First, in autoimmune liver diseases anti-GOR is only found in autoimmune hepatitis type 2b, i.e. in LKM-1 antibody positive patients that are HCV positive [5]. In addition, anti-GOR are only found in chronic hepatitis D if these patients show HCV superinfection, i.e. are anti-HCV and HCV RNA positive [21].

Little is known about the nature of the GOR antigen. It is a nuclear antigen and its expression seems to be particularly high in tumour tissue of hepatocellular carcinoma [22]. In this context, it is of particular interest that we could generate GOR specific T cell clones from a patient with hepatocellular carcinoma and chronic hepatitis C [23]. In the meantime a second GOR epitope was identified on the GOR cDNA sequence that is also recognized by antibodies in sera from patients with HCV infection (Mishiro *et al.*, personal communication). Our data were all obtained with a specific ELISA based on the synthetic GOR-2 epitope [5].

It is being discussed whether anti-GOR antibodies are true autoantibodies that persist once they are induced by HCV or whether they rather reflect cross-reaction betweeen HCV and self sequences. There is some molecular homology between GOR and the sequence of HCV core peptide. Possibly anti-GOR antibodies just reflect a specific anti-HCV antibody cross-reacting between HCV and self components. This could be supported by our observation that anti-GOR antibody titers decline if interferon treatment in hepatitis C is effective [24]. However, Japanese investigators could not confirm this observation [25].

Hepatitis C virus, mixed cryoglobulinemia and liver disease

Reports from Italy [26], France [27] and lately the United States [28] have indicated the association of HCV infection with a significant proportion of patients with type II and type III mixed cryoglobulinemia [29]. HCV-RNA was detected in up to 90 % of such cases while anti-HCV positivity in serum by commercial ELISAs (HCV peptides c22-3, c33,

C-100 and 5-1-1) was significantly lower [29]. Since HCV RNA was described as a significant component of the cryoprecipitates, it may be speculated whether other anti-HCV antibodies than those detected in the commercial ELISAs are responsible for the formation of these cryoprecipitates. Interestingly these patients seem to profit from interferon treament [29]. This is interesting since in the past severe cases with this syndrome were treated with plasmapheresis, corticosteroids and cytotoxic drugs like cyclophosphamide. Concerning autoimmune phenomena in this HCV associated syndrome, we observed antinuclear, smooth muscle but no liver-kidney microsomal antibodies (Ferri *et al.*, unpublished data). It will be interesting to see the evaluation of the fine specificity of anti-HCV antibodies in these patients, HCV genotyping and immunogenetic analysis. It has to be evaluated whether liver involvement in these HCV associated cases with mixed cryoglobulinemia is due to chronic HCV infection, deposition of immune complexes in liver tissue or associated autoimmune liver disease.

Membranoproliferative glomerulonephritis and hepatitis C

Very recently, eight patients were described suffering from membranoproliferative glomerulonephritis associated with hepatitis C virus infection [30]. All patients had proteinuria, seven decreased renal function. Renal biopsy revealed membranoproliferative glomerulonephritis characterized by the deposition of IgG, IgM and C3 in glomeruli. All patients had HCV-RNA in serum, elevated transaminases, hypocomplementemia and the majority had cryoglobulins. Cryoprecipitates contained HCV-RNA and IgG anti-HCV to the nucleocapsid core HCV antigen (c22-3) as well as IgM rheumatoid factor. All four patients who were treated with interferon alpha 2b decreased HCV replication, improved renal function and liver disease [30]. It is concluded from these studies that HCV infection was involved in the induction of membranoproliferative glomerulonephritis in these patients. Open questions are how often glomerulonephritis occurs as a consequence of chronic HCV infection and whether interferon has a beneficial long-term effect in these patients. Presumably more cases of membranoproliferative glomerulonephritis associated with HCV infection will be published in the future. This information at least adds to our understanding of the interaction between hepatitis C virus and the immune system.

Porphyria cutanea tarda and hepatitis C virus infection

Porphyria cutanea tarda has also been linked to HCV infection [31]. However, much more information is necessary to understand the mechanisms by which HCV may induce porphyria cutanea tarda, in particular whether the immune system is involved. Own data resulting from a collaboration with an Italian group of investigators (Ferri *et al.*, unpublished data) show that some of the HCV associated cases with porphyria cutanea tarda in contrast to HCV associated mixed cryoglobulinemia are positive for LKM_1 antibodies in serum, an autoantibody known to be induced by HCV infection.

Sjögren'syndrome

Several reports indicate that Sjögren's syndrome at least in geographical areas with a high prevalence of HCV infection may be associated with HCV infection [29]. Sjögren's syndrome is also regarded as a syndrome of autoimmune background where the immune attack targets the epithelium of salivary and lacrimal glands. Antinuclear SSA/La antibodies are indicators of a disturbed immune system and specific diagnostic markers for Sjögren's syndrome. It seems possible that HCV by infecting the epithelium of salivary and lacrymal glands leads to the sicca syndrome. We need more information such as the expression of HCV proteins and or HCV-RNA in these epithelia before we understand the involvement of HCV in the pathogenesis of Sjögren's syndrome. Furthermore it will be interesting to evaluate differences in the autoimmune serological markers between HCV positive and negative patients with Sjögren's syndrome.

References

1. Esteban JL, Esteban R, Viladomiu L, *et al.* Hepatitis C virus antibodies among risk groups in Spain. Lancet 1989 ; 2 : 294-7.
2. McFarlane IG, Smith HM, Johnson PJ, Bray GP, Vergani D, Williams R. Hepatitis C virus antibodies in chronic active hepatitis : pathogenetic factor or false-positive result ? Lancet 1990 ; 335 : 754-7.
3. Nishioka M. Nuclear antigens in autoimmune hepatitis. In : Meyer zum Büschenfelde KH, Manns MP, Hoofnagle JR, eds. Immunology and the Liver. Lancester, England : MTP Press LTD, 1993.
4. Lenzi M, Johnson PJ, McFarlane IG, *et al.* Antibodies to hepatitis C virus in autoimmune liver disease ; evidence for geographical heterogeneity. Lancet 1991 ; 338 : 1370-8.
5. Michel G, Ritter A, Gerken G, *et al.* Anti GOR and hepatitis C virus in autoimmune liver disease. Lancet 1992 ; 339 : 267-9.

6. Lunel F, Abuaf N, Frangeul L, Grippon P, Perrin M, Le Coz Y, Valla D, *et al.* Liver/kidney microsome antibody type 1 and hepatitis C virus infection. Hepatology 1992 ; 16 : 630-6.
7. Miyachi K. Personal communication, 1992.
8. Czaja A, Manns MP, Homburger H. Frequency and significance of antibodies to liver/kidney microsome type 1 in adults with chronic active hepatitis. Gastroenterology 1992 ; 103 : 1290-5.
9. Homberg JC, Abuaf N, Bernard O, *et al.* Chronic active hepatitis associated with anti-liver/kidney microsome autoantibody type I : a second type of « autoimmune hepatitis ». Hepatology 1987 ; 1 : 1333-9.
10. Sacher M, Blümel P, Thaler H, Manns M. Chronic active hepatitis associated with vitiligo, nail dystrophy, alopecia and a new variant of LKM antibodies. J Hepatol 1990 ; 10 : 364-9.
11. Manns MP, Scheucher S, Jentzsch M, *et al.* Genetics in autoimmune hepatitis type 2. Hepatology 1991 ; 14 : 60A.
12. Lenzi M, Mantovani W, Cataleta M, Basllardini G, Cassani F, Giostra F, Muratori L, Bianchi FB. HLA typing in autoimmune hepatitis (AI-CAH) type 2. J Hepatol 1992 ; 16 : 59.
13. Ruiz-Moreno M, Rua JA, Carreno V, *et al.* Autoimmune chronic active hepatitis type 2 manifested during interferon therapy in children. J Hepatol 1991 ; 12 : 265-6.
14. Vento S, di Perri G, Luzzati R, *et al.* Type 2 autoimmune hepatitis and hepatitis C virus infection. Lancet 1990 ; 335 : 921-2.
15. Zanger UM, Hauri HP, Loeper J, *et al.* Antibodies against human cytochrome P450 db 1 in autoimmune hepatitis type II. Proc Natl Acad Sci USA 1988 ; 27 : 8256-60.
16. Manns M, Johnson EF, Griffin KJ, *et al.* The major target antigen of liver kidney microsomal autoantibodies in idiopathic autoimmune hepatitis is cytochrome P450 db1. J Clin Invest 1989 ; 83 : 1066-72.
17. Manns M, Griffin KJ, Sullivan KF, *et al.* LKM-1 autoantibodies recognize a short linear sequence in P450 II D6. J Clin Invest 1991 ; 88 : 1370-8.
18. Ma Y, Lenzi M, Gäken J, Thomas MG, Farzaneh F, Ballardini G, Cassani F, Mieli-Vergani G, Bianchi FB, Vergani D. The target antigen of liver kidney microsomal antibody is different in type II autoimmune chronic active hepatitis and chronic hepatitis C virus infection. J Hepatol 1992 ; 16 : 4.
19. Durazzo M, Philipp T, Lüttig B, Loges S, Schmidt E, Rizzetto M, Manns MP. Heterogeneity of microsomal autoantibodies (LKM) in chronic hepatitis C virus (HCV) infection. Falk Symposium n° 70, Immunology and the Liver, 1992 : 12.
20. Mishiro S, Hoshi Y, Takeda K, *et al.* Non A, non B hepatitis specific antibodies directed at host-derived epitope : implication for an autoimmune process. Lancet 1990 ; 2 : 1400-3.
21. Durazzo M, Michel G, Philipp T, Braun HB, Lüttig B, Rizzetto M, Manns M. Anti-GOR in hepatitis D : specific association with hepatitis C virus superinfection. Hepatology 1992 ; 16 : 76A.
22. Mishiro S, Takeda K, Hoshi Y, Yoshikawa A, Gotanda T, Itoh Y. An autoantibody crossreactive to hepatitis C virus core and host nuclear antigen. Autoimmunity 1991 10 : 269-73.
23. Rehermann B, Schneider S, Michel G, Manns MP. GOR-spezifische T-Lymphozyten : Proliferation bei chronischer Hepatitis C. Z Gastroenterol 1993 ; 31 : 84.
24. Mergener K, Michel G, Braun HB, Thome-Kromer B, Korn A, Müller R, Manns M. Anti-GOR titers in chronic hepatitis C in relation to interferon therapy. J Hepatol 1992 ; 16 : 4.
25. Lau JYN, Davis GL, Orito E, Qian KP, Mizokami M. Significance of antibody to the host cellular gene derived epitope GOR in chronic hepatitis C virus infection. J Hepatol 1993 ; 17 : 253-7.
26. Ferri C, Greco F, Longombardo G., *et al.* Association between hepatitis C virus in patients with mixed cryoglobulinemia. Arthritis Rheum 1991 ; 34 : 1606-10.

27. Lunel F, Musset L, Caboub P, Perrin M, Frangeul L, Bousquet O, Godeau P, Valla D, Le Charpentier Y, Opolon P, Huraux JM. Prevalence of mixed cryoglobulinemia in 112 patients with viral and non viral chronic hepatitis or cirrhosis.J Hepatol 1992 ; 16 : 13.
28. Agnello V, Chung RT, Kaplan L. A role for hepatitis C virus infection in type II cryoglobulinemia. N Engl J Med 1992 ; 19 : 1490.
29. Bloch KJ. Cryoglobulinemia and hepatitis C virus. N Engl J Med 1992 ; 327 : 1521.
30. Johnson RJ, Gretch DR, Yamabe H, Hart J, Bacchi CE, Hartwell P, Couser W, Corey L, Wener MH, Alpers C, Wilson R. Membranoproliferative glomerulonephritis associated with hepatitis C virus infection. N Engl J Med 1993 ; 18 : 465-70.
31. Fargion S, Piperno A, Capellini MD, Sampietro M, Fracanzani AL, Romano R, Caldarelli R, Marcelli R, Vecchi L, Fiorelli G. Hepatitis C virus and porphyria cutanea tarda : evidence of a strong association. Hepatology 1992 ; 16 : 1322-3.

Progress in Hepatology 93. J.P. Miguet and D. Dhumeaux, eds.
John Libbey Eurotext, Paris © 1993, pp. 89-97

10

Therapy of chronic hepatitis B and C

J. H. HOOFNAGLE

Division of Digestive Diseases and Nutrition, National Institute of Diabetes and Digestive and Kidney Diseases, National Institutes of Health, Bethesda, MD 28092, USA.

Alpha-interferon is now licensed for use in both chronic hepatitis B and C. However, interferon therapy is far from satisfactory. Four issues warrant discussion : *a*) the optimal dose and regimen of alpha interferon for each disease ; *b*) indications for therapy ; *c*) the definition of a response ; *d*) management of the patient who does not respond or who relapses when therapy is stopped.

Chronic hepatitis B

Optimal regimen of alpha-interferon

A 4 to 6 month course of alpha-interferon is effective in inducing a long-term remission in disease in 25 % to 40 % of patients with chronic hepatitis B [1-3]. The correct dose of alpha-interferon is 4 to 5 mu given daily or 9 to 10 mu given three times weekly. This is a higher dose than what is used in chronic hepatitis C (3 mu three times weekly) ; but this higher dose is necessary for optimal effect. The only exception to this is the patient with decompensated cirrhosis. In addition, treatment for 4 to 6 months is adequate ; more prolonged courses have not been found to improve the response rate in chronic hepatitis B.

Criteria for therapy

Interferon is recommended for patients with persistent elevations in serum aminotransferases , HBsAg, HBeAg and HBV DNA in serum, and well compensated liver disease with no other complicating illness. These criteria are somewhat restrictive but important.

First, aminotransferase should be elevated. Alpha-interferon has little effect in patients who are healthy HBsAg carriers or who have normal alanine aminotransferase (ALT) levels [2, 5]. The response rate to interferon correlates with the initial ALT level. Patients with chronic hepatitis B with ALT levels less than twice the upper limit of normal rarely respond and probably should be monitored without therapy.

Second, HBsAg, HBeAg and HBV DNA should be present in serum ; therapy is ineffective in patients without active viral replication. Some patients, however, have HBV DNA in serum without HBeAg. These patients have a strain of virus with a mutation in the pre-core region of the HBV genome which allows for viral replication but blocks synthesis of HBeAg [4]. Three randomized controlled trials of alpha-interferon in patients with the HBeAg-minus mutant have shown that therapy is effective, but perhaps less so than in HBeAg positive patients [4-6]. Relapses after therapy are also common.

Third, patients should have well-compensated liver disease. This is defined by the absence of ascites, hepatic encephalopathy, variceal hemorrhage, persistent jaundice (bilirubin greater than 7oμmol/l) or wasting. Dramatic beneficial responses have been noted in about 35 % of these patients [7, 8], but side effects are common and severe and a sustained response is unlikely if the disease is too far advanced (Child's class C). Therapy should be started at doses of 1 to 2 mu three times weekly and increased based upon tolerance. Patients need to be monitored carefully for side effects especially bacterial infections, psychiatric complications, and worsening of the liver disease. These patients should only be treated by physicians with extensive experience in using interferon and in managing patients with hepatic failure.

Finally, therapy should be limited to patients without other severe complicating illnesses. Most important in this respect is immunodeficiency or immunosuppression which can block the effects of alpha-interferon. Thus, in patients with solid organ transplants, interferon has little effect and long-term responses to treatment are rare [9]. Patients with established

AIDS and severe immune deficiency also do not usually respond to interferon therapy, although patients with anti-HIV and normal levels of $CD4^+$ cells appear to respond normally [2].

Two other situations in treating HBV related disease warrant comment : acute hepatitis B and children. Alpha-interferon is not indicated in acute hepatitis B as clinical trials have not shown improvement in the course of disease or prevention of chronicity with therapy. Alpha-interferon has not been extensively studied in children with chronic hepatitis B, although small trials suggest that they respond to treatment at a rate similar to that in adults [3, 10]. The dose of alpha-interferon in children should be 4 to 6 mu/m^2 three times weekly for four to six months.

Definition of a response

A response to alpha-interferon is marked by the loss of HBV DNA (and HBeAg if present) from the serum and improvement in clinical disease. Typically, HBeAg becomes negative and ALT falls after rather than during interferon therapy. HBsAg also becomes undetectable in many patients who lose HBeAg, but generally months to years after therapy [11].

A beneficial response to alpha-interferon should include the following elements : *a*) loss of HBV DNA from serum (as measured by direct blot or liquid hybridization) within 6 months, *b*) loss of HBeAg from serum (if present initially), and *c*) fall of ALT into the normal range or to within 1.5 times the upper limit of the normal range within one year of starting therapy.

Non-responders

A common and difficult problem in chronic hepatitis B is the management of patients who fail to respond to an adequate course of alpha-interferon treatment. These patients rarely benefit from retreatment and should be followed without therapy. In these patients, other approaches to therapy are being actively investigated [12]. The development of animal models of HBV infection and cell culture systems for studying replication have provided the tools to screen large numbers of antiviral substances. Agents currently under evaluation include thymosin, levamisole, interleukin 2, gamma-interferon, granulocyte-macrophage colony stimulating factor, gancyclovir, dideoxyinosine, ribavirin, and newer nucleoside analogues including fluoro-iodo-arabinofuranosyl-uracil (FIAU), 3'-thia-fluorocytosine (FTC), 3-thia-cytidine (3TC), famciclovir and the carbocyclic analogue of 2' deoxyguanosine (2-CDG) [12-14]. These nucleoside analogues are well absorbed orally and have been shown to have activity *in vitro* and *in vivo* against HBV, but have yet to be proven effective in inducing remissions in chronic hepatitis B at a rate higher than what occurs spontaneously. Furthermore, their short and long-term toxicities remain to be defined. Other advances in molecular biology and immunotherapy have also provided potentially valuable, innovative approaches to therapy, such as use of antisense oligonucleotides, ribozymes against HBV RNA, monoclonal antibodies to HBsAg, and HBV antigen-specific immunocyte transfer [15]. These advances indicate that a rational, safe and effective therapy for chronic hepatitis B may soon be available.

Chronic hepatitis C

Optimal regimen of alpha-interferon

A six-month course of alpha-interferon in doses of 2 to 5 mu thrice weekly is followed by a fall of ALT into the normal range and improvement in liver histology in at least 50 % of patients with chronic hepatitis C [16-19]. The decreases in ALT levels are accompanied by a fall in HCV RNA levels in blood and liver ; most patients who respond become HCV RNA negative [20]. Unfortunately, a high proportion of patients who respond to therapy relapse once it is stopped. Relapses are marked by a return of serum HCV RNA and ALT elevations. Thus, long-term beneficial responses occur in only 20 % to 30 % of patients.

At present, the recommended regimen of therapy is 3 mu given thrice weekly for six months. Lower doses are clearly less effective [17]. Higher doses are currently being evaluated [21, 22]. There is some evidence, however, that doses of 5 mu three times weekly and regimens of therapy for 12 months provide a higher rate of long-term responses [16, 21], but at present they must be considered experimental.

Criteria for therapy

Alpha-interferon is currently recommended for patients with well-compensated chronic hepatitis C, persistently raised ALT levels, chronic hepatitis by liver biopsy and serologic or epidemiologic evidence of HCV infection (anti-HCV or a history of exposure before onset of hepatitis). Analysis of predictive factors for a long-term response suggests that patients without cirrhosis and with a relatively short duration of disease are most likely to benefit [23]. Thus, therapy needs not be restricted to patients with severe disease, although it is inadvisable to treat patients with normal ALT levels or minimal disease.

Other patients who deserve consideration for interferon therapy inlcude patients with **acute hepatitis C**, children, patients with atypical serology, or decompensated cirrhosis or immunodeficiency. A high percentage of patients with acute hepatitis C develop chronic hepatitis. Four controlled trials of alpha-interferon in acute post-transfusion hepatitis (largely hepatitis C) have been published [24-27]. In all four trials, a higher percentage of treated than untreated patients had normal ALT levels after 1 to 2 years of follow-up (57 % to 64 % *versus* 11 % to 42 %). However, the differences were not great making recommendations for treatment difficult. Patients can recover spontaneously without treatment ; thus, therapy is best restricted to patients who have evidence of developing chronic infection. Persistence of ALT elevations and HCV RNA in serum for two months after onset of acute hepatitis C is a reasonable guideline for initiation of therapy with alpha-interferon. At that point, it is appropriate to use the same regimen of interferon as is recommended for chronic hepatitis C.

Preliminary reports indicate that the response rates of **children** with chronic hepatitis C are similar to those in adults [28]. Treatment is recommended in doses of 3 mu/m^2 three times weekly for 24 weeks. Some patients with chronic hepatitis C have **atypical serologic results** and test negative for anti-HCV by currently available immunoassays. Important diagnoses to exclude are autoimmune hepatitis, drug-induced liver injury, sclerosing cholangitis, Wilson's disease and alpha 1-antitrypsin deficiency. In some cases the diagnosis of chronic hepatitis C can be established by research assays for HCV RNA in serum or HCV antigen in liver. In other cases, however, the diagnosis remains elusive and the severity of disease warrants treatment. There is a need for caution in using interferon in this situation, because patients with autoimmune hepatitis can exhibit a severe worsening with treatment. For this reason, it is appropriate to try first a course of corticosteroids in patients in whom a specific diagnosis cannot be made. If there is no response, a trial of interferon is warranted.

There have been few studies of therapy of patients with **clinically apparent cirrhosis** due to hepatitis C. These patients can respond to interferon but they are particularly susceptible to side effects and have a high rate of relapse after treatment. As in chronic hepatitis B, only patients with early or mildly decompensated cirrhosis should be treated. For advanced cases, liver transplantation offers the only possibility for a sustained improvement in health. Patients with **immune deficiencies** are frequently infected with HCV, and the immunosuppression itself may worsen the liver disease. Pilot studies have suggested that patients with a combination of HCV and HIV infection can respond to alpha-interferon therapy as can patients with recurrent hepatitis C after liver transplantation with decreases in viral replication and ALT levels [9, 29]. The safety and relative benefit of interferon therapy in these situations is still unclear and these patients should not receive interferon outside of controlled trials.

Definition of response

Four patterns of response to alpha-interferon therapy of chronic hepatitis C can be defined. Approximately 25 % of patients have a **sustained beneficial response** : ALT levels begin to fall within the first months of treatment and are often normal by two to three months. Serum levels of HCV RNA usually fall with the decrease in ALT, and both ALT and HCV RNA remain normal or undetectable after therapy. Another 25 % of patients have a complete response while on interferon but promptly **relapse** when treatment is stopped. These patients may become negative for HCV RNA on treatment, but redevelop this viral marker when interferon is stopped and ALT levels rise. A third group consists of about 25 % of the patients who have **a partial or transient response** only, in whom ALT levels decrease but do not become normal or become normal only transiently (breakthrough) and then rise despite continuation of interferon. ALT levels may decrease into the normal range if the dose of interferon is increased, but not all patients will be able to tolerate the increased side effects that accompany the higher dose. A final 25 % of patients have **no response** to interferon ; ALT levels remain elevated and serum HCV RNA present throughout treatment. A long-term response to interferon is defined as persistence of normal ALT levels for a year after therapy. Longer follow-up is available on few patients. In one study, 3 to 6 year follow-up showed that patients continued to have normal ALT levels and no HCV RNA [30]. In a second study, late relapses were described and not all patients with a sustained response continued to be HCV RNA negative [31].

Non-responders

There is little information regarding the efficacy of retreatment or use of higher doses of alpha-interferon in patients who do not respond to treatment or in those who relapse when therapy. Retreatment should be advised only for those patients who had a beneficial response to an initial course of therapy with few side effects but who subsequently relapsed and use of higher doses of interferon in a more prolonged course is advisable. A patient who has absolutely no response to interferon during an initial course of therapy should not be retreated. These patients are excellent candidates for future trials of other antiviral agents. They should also be carefully evaluated for the possibility of having another form of liver disease, perhaps autoimmune or alcoholic hepatitis.

Pilot studies of other antiviral agents that might be used alone or in combination with interferon in chronic hepatitis C have recently been initiated. The most promising such antiviral agent is ribavirin. Ribavirin has a broad range of activity against several DNA and RNA viruses *in vitro*. It is well absorbed orally and relatively safe, its only side effect being hemolysis. In two pilot studies, a six-month course of ribavirin therapy was found to lead to a decrease in ALT in the majority of patients with chronic hepatitis C [32, 33]. Unfortunately, the improvements in ALT were not accompanied by major improvements in liver histology or HCV RNA levels. Randomized controlled trials of ribavirin and the combination of ribavirin with interferon are now underway.

Few other antiviral agents have been evaluated in patients with chronic hepatitis C. Future advances in therapy of chronic hepatitis C would be benefitted most by development of reliable tissue culture systems for evaluating HCV replication and the effect of antiviral agents [34].

References

1. Perrillo RP, Schiff ER, Davis GL, *et al.* A randomized controlled trial of interferon alfa-2b alone and after prednisone withdrawal for the treatment of chronic hepatitis B. N Engl J Med 1990 ; 323 : 295-301.
2. Hoofnagle JH, Peters MG, Mullen KD, *et al.* Randomized controlled trial of a four-month course of recombinant human alpha interferon in chronic type B hepatitis. Gastroenterology 1988 ; 95 : 1318-25.
3. Lok ASF, Wu PC, Lai CL, *et al.* A controlled trial of interferon with or without prednisone priming for chronic hepatitis B. Gastroenterology 1992 ; 102 : 2091-7.
4. Brunetto MR, Oliveri F, Rocca G, *et al.* Natural course and response to interferon of chronic hepatitis B accompanied by antibody to hepatitis e antigen. Hepatology 1989 ; 10 : 198-202.
5. Hadziyannis S, Bramou T, Makris A, *et al.* Interferon alpha-2b treatment of HBeAg negative/serum HBV DNA positive chronic active hepatitis type B. J Hepatol 1990 ; 11 : S133-6.
6. Fattovich G, Farci P, Brollo L, *et al.* A randomized controlled trial of lymphoblastoid interferon-alpha in patients with chronic hepatitis B lacking HBeAg. Hepatology 1992 ; 15 : 584-9.
7. Hoofnagle JH, Di Bisceglie AM, Waggoner JG, Park Y. Interferon alfa for patients with

clinically apparent cirrhosis due to chronic hepatitis B. Gastroenterology 1993 ; 104 : 1116-21.
8. Perrillo R, Tamburro C, Regenstein F, *et al.* Treatment of decompensated chronic hepatitis B (CHB) with a titratable, low dose regimen of recombinant interferon alfa-2b (rIFN a-2b). Hepatology 1992 ; 16 : 126A [abstract].
9. Wright HI, Gavaler JS, Van Thiel DH. Preliminary experience with alpha-2b interferon therapy of viral hepatitis in liver allograft recipients. Transplantation 1992 ; 53 : 121-4.
10. Ruiz-Moreno M, Rua MJ, Molina J, *et al.* Prospective, randomized controlled trial of interferon-alpha in children with chronic hepatitis B. Hepatology 1991 ; 13 : 1035-9.
11. Korenman J, Baker B, Waggoner J, *et al.* Long-term remission in chronic hepatitis B after alpha-interferon therapy. Ann Intern Med 1991 ; 114 : 629-34.
12. Hoofnagle JH, Di Bisceglie AM. Antiviral therapy of viral hepatitis. In : Galasso GJ, Whitley RJ, Merigan TC, eds. Antiviral agents and viral diseases of man. 3rd edition. New York : Raven Press, 1990 : 415-59.
13. Fried M, Di Bisceglie AM, Straus SE, Savarese B, Beames MP, Hoofnagle JH. FIAU, a new oral anti-viral agent, profoundly inhibits HBV DNA in patients with chronic hepatitis B. Hepatology 1992 : 16 : 127A abstract.
14. Furman PA, Davis M, Liotta DC, *et al.* The anti-hepatitis B virus activities, cytotoxicities, and anabolic profiles of the (−) and (+) enantiomers of cis-5-fluoro-1-[2-(hydroxymethyl)-1,3-oxathiolan-5-yl] cytosine. Antimicrob Agents Chemother 1992 ; 35 : 2686-92.
15. Lok ASF, Liang RHS, Chung HT. Recovery from chronic hepatitis B. Ann Intern Med 1982 ; 116 : 957 [letter].
16. Hoofnagle JH, Mullen KD, Jones DB, *et al.* Treatment of chronic non-A, non-B hepatitis with recombinant human alpha interferon : a preliminary report. N Engl J Med 1986 ; 315 : 1575-8.
17. Davis GL, Balart LA, Schiff ER, *et al.* Treatment of chronic hepatitis C with recombinant interferon alfa : a multicenter randomized, controlled trial. N Engl J Med 1989 ; 321 : 1501-5.
18. Di Bisceglie AM, Martin P, Kassianides C, *et al.* Recombinant interferon alfa therapy for chronic hepatitis C : a randomized, double-blind, placebo-controlled trial. N Engl J Med 1989 ; 321 : 1506-10.
19. Marcellin P, Boyer N, Giostra E, *et al.* Recombinant human alpha-interferon in patients with chronic non-A, non-B hepatitis : a multicenter randomized controlled trial from France. Hepatology 1991 ; 13 : 393-7.
20. Shindo M, Di Bisceglie AM, Cheung L, *et al.* Decrease in serum hepatitis C viral RNA during alpha-interferon therapy for chronic hepatitis C. Ann Intern Med 1991 ; 115 : 700-4.
21. Alberti A, Chemello L, Diodati G, *et al.* Treatment of chronic hepatitis C with different regimens of interferon alpha-2a (IFN-2a). Hepatology 1992 ; 16 : 75A [abstract].
22. Craxi A, Di Marco V, Lo Iacono O, *et al.* Lymphoblastoid alpha-interferon for post-transfusion chronic hepatitis C : a randomized trial of 6 vs 12 months treatment. J Hepatol 1992 ; 16 : S8 [abstract].
23. Camma C, Craxi A, Tine F, *et al.* Predictors of response to alpha-interferon (IFN) in chronic hepatitis C : a multivariate analysis on 361 treated patients. Hepatology 1992 ; 16 : 131A [abstract].
24. Omata M, Yokosuka O, Takano S, *et al.* Resolution of acute hepatitis C after therapy with natural beta interferon. Lancet 1991 ; 338 : 914-5.
25. Alberti A, Chemello L, Benvegnu L, *et al.* Pilot study of interferon alpha-2a therapy in preventing chronic evolution of acute hepatitis C. In : Hollinger RB, Lemon S, Margolis H, eds. Viral hepatitis and liver disease. Baltimore : Williams and Wilkins, 1991 : 656-8.
26. Viladomiu L, Gonzalez A, Lopez-Talavera JC, *et al.* A randomized controlled trial of alpha-interferon in acute posttransfusion C hepatitis. J Hepatol 1990 ; 11 : S64 [abstract].
27. Rumi MG, Lampertico P, Soffredini R, *et al.* Serum HCV-RNA in patients with acute hepatitis C treated with recombinant interferon alfa. Hepatology 1992 ; 16 : 72A [abstract].
28. Ruiz-Moreno M, Rua MJ, Castillo I, *et al.* Treatment of children with chronic hepatitis

C with chronic hepatitis C with recombinant interferon-alpha : a pilot study. Hepatology 1992 ; 16 : 882-5.
29. Wright TL, Ferrell L, Lake J, *et al.* Hepatitis C viral RNA in patients on interferon (IFN)-alpha for post-liver transplant (OLTx) hepatitis. Gastroenterology 1992 ; 102 : A910 [abstract].
30. Shindo M, Di Bisceglie AM, Hoofnagle JH. Long-term follow-up of patients with chronic hepatitis C treated with alpha interferon. Hepatology 1992 ; 15 : 1013-6.
31. Marcellin P, Boyer N, Martinot-Peignoux M, *et al.* Detection of serum HCV RNA by polymerase chain reaction (PCR) in patients with chronic hepatitis C with sustained response to recombinant alpha interferon. J Hepatol 1992 ; 16 : S8 [abstract].
32. Reichard O, Andersson J, Schvarcz R, Weiland O. Ribavirin treatment for chronic hepatitis C. Lancet 1991 ; 337 : 1058-61.
33. Di Bisceglie AM, Shindo M, Fong TL, *et al.* A pilot study of ribavirin therapy for chronic hepatitis C. Hepatology 1992 ; 16 : 649-54.
34. Shimizu YK, Iwamoto A, Hijikata M, *et al.* Evidence for *in vitro* replication of hepatitis C virus genome in a human T cell line. Proc Natl Acad Sci USA 1992 ; 89 : 5477-81.

Progress in Hepatology 93. J.P. Miguet and D. Dhumeaux, eds.
John Libbey Eurotext, Paris © 1993, pp. 99-107

11

Future therapy for B virus chronic hepatitis

M. THURSZ, H. THOMAS

Department of Medicine, St Mary's Hospital Medical School, London W2 1PG, England.

Great advances have been made over the last two decades in our knowledge of the biology of hepatitis B virus (HBV) and the immunological response to the virus in both acute and chronic infection. However, the best available therapy for chronic HBV infection elicits a successful response in only about 40 % of patients [1]. Nevertheless, control of HBV should still be seen as an attainable goal as new anti-viral therapies are emerging and our understanding of viral immunology will soon be translated into new therapeutic modalities. There are two broad methods of treatment which we will discuss here : the first is the control of viral replication by pharmacological means and the second is the application of specific immune components as therapeutic tools. Finally, we will discuss the way in which these therapies might be deployed in different patient groups.

Control of viral replication

Dideoxynucleoside analogues

Recent attempts to inhibit viral replication pharmacologically have focused on the inhibition of the reverse transcriptase encoded by HBV. A group of dideoxynucleoside analogues have been developed with the aim of selectively inhibiting the reverse transcriptase (RT) of HIV and also possibly HBV ; these include 2', 3'-dideoxyadenosine (ddA), 2', 3'-dideoxycytosine (ddC), 2', 3'-dideoxyguanosine (ddG), adenosine arabinoside (araA), cytosine arabinoside (araC) and AZT. AZT and ddA are both potent inhibitors of the HIV RT and have been used successfully in the clinical setting, however neither drug has any significant action on HBV RT [2]. AraA and araC are both potent inhibitors of HBV polymerase and RT. AraA has been tested clinically in patients with chronic HBV infection but the outcome was poor due to toxic side effects which precluded therapy of satisfactory duration and dose [3] ; araC is more toxic than araA.

Toxicity of these compounds is manifest predominantly as myelosuppression and neuropathy and is thought to arise from the inhibition of mammalian DNA polymerases. Mitochondrial damage secondary to the inhibition of DNA polymerase gamma has been implicated in the nerve lesions seen with use of dideoxynucleoside analogues. 3 Thiacytidine (3TC) is a new dideoxynucleoside analogue which potently inhibits HBV RT but probably not HBV polymerase. The enantiomers of this compound can be separated and it is found that, although both enantiomers inhibit RT, the (-) enantiomer does not inhibit polymerase and is therefore far less cytotoxic [4]. Consequently, HBeAg persists in patient serum despite the cessation of viral replication and fall in HBV DNA (Figure 1).

3TC was originally developed as a potential anti-HIV agent but during clinical trials which included patients co-infected with HBV it was found that HBV replication was markedly inhibited. Initial results confirm the lack of toxicity of 3TC and clinical trials in patients with chronic HBV are currently underway.

Famciclovir

Acyclovir and other compounds of similar structure are effective against the herpes viruses and at high doses it is known that acyclovir will inhibit replication of hepatitis B. Herpes viruses encode an enzyme with thymidine kinase activity which selectively concentrates the active drug within the infected cell. Despite the fact that HBV is not known to possess such an enzyme it was found that acyclovir inhibits replication of HBV in cell culture [5] and inhibits replication of duck hepatitis virus in the Pekin duck model [6].

Famciclovir is a drug from the same family as acyclovir which is significantly more potent. Famciclovir is a pro-drug which is converted to penciclovir on absorption through the gastrointestinal tract. In herpes infected cells the drug is phosphorylated by the virally encoded thymidine kinase whereas in normal cells drug levels equilibrate with plasma. In this way the active drug can be concentrated by a factor of five in the infected cells. The phosphorylated drug inhibits viral DNA polymerase thus blocking the synthesis of viral DNA. The mechanism of action on HBV is unknown. In our own study significant inhibition of HBV replication was seen in 5 out of 6 patients treated for 10 days with 250 mg tds of famciclovir (unpublished results). Further clinical studies are underway.

It would be reasonable to hypothesise that inhibition of viral replication would reduce the expression of viral peptides in association with MHC class I molecules. However, experimental evidence shows that acyclovir increases class I expression on the infected hepatocyte, which suggests that viral replication per se inhibits class I expression [7].

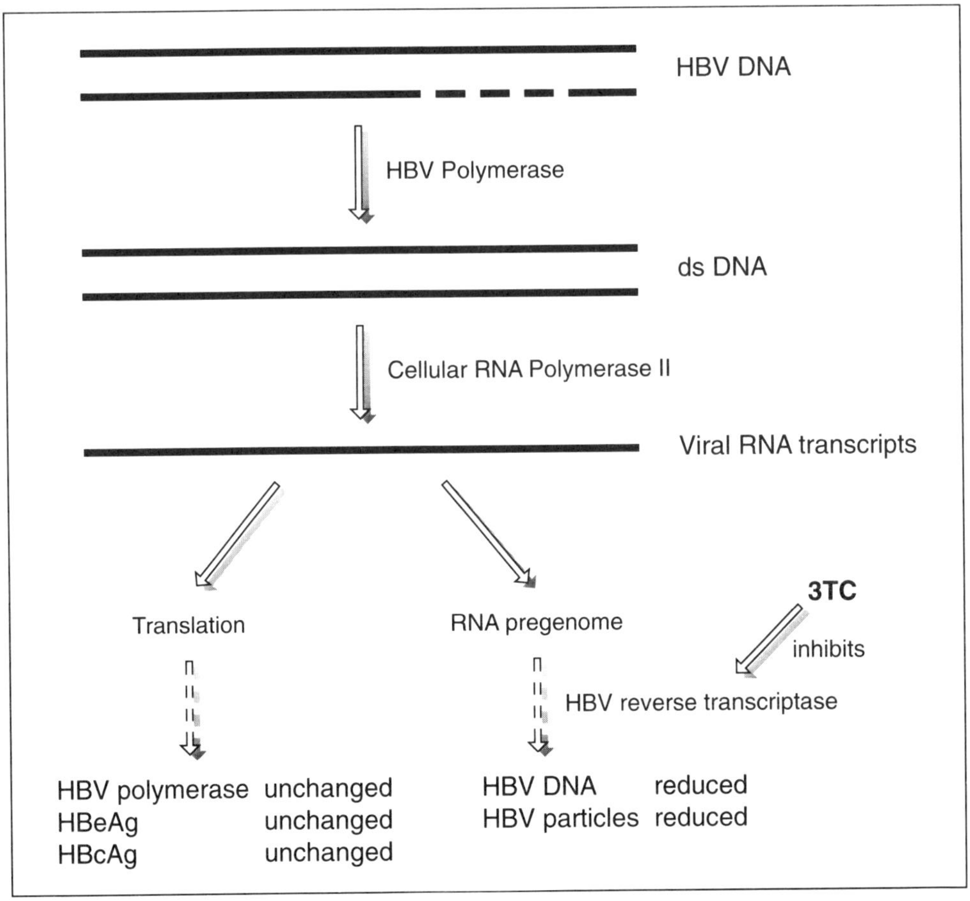

Figure 1. Mechanism of action of 3 thiacytidine.

Immunotherapy (Figure 2)

Enhancement of antigen presentation

Immunological recognition of virus and virally infected cells depends on the presentation of foreign proteins as oligopeptide epitopes in the clefts of HLA class I and II molecules. These epitope/MHC combinations are recognized by complementary T cell receptors on the cell surfaces of $CD4^+$ and $CD8^+$ T lymphocytes. This antigen presentation is accompanied by a series of accessory interactions between cell surface macromolecules which may determine the nature of the response to antigen recognition. At the chemical level the interaction between these molecules is ascribed to the formation of Schiff bases (transient carbonyl-amino condensations). Cell surface Schiff base formation can be enhanced up to 100 fold by incubation with galactose oxidase (GO) and neuraminidase (NA). NAGO has been used experimentally as an adjuvant for immunization and has been shown to greatly potentiate proliferative and antibody responses [8]. An orally active agent has been developed which has the same effect as NAGO and will soon be subjected to clinical trials in an animal model.

Adoptive transfer of lymphocytes

Adoptive transfer of immune effector cells has been used for many years to explore the cell mediated immunology of certain diseases. It has been shown that lesional lymphocytes from a diseased animal will induce the same disease when transferred to a previously healthy syngeneic animal [9]. In chronic hepatitis B the components of the cellular immune system are pivotal in the disease process. Whereas HBc-specific $CD8^+$ cytotoxic T cells (CTL), which are thought to be responsible for clearance of infected hepatocytes, are detectable in peripheral blood in the acute infection, these cells are not found in patients with chronic infection [10]. Moreover the magnitude of the $CD4^+$ lymphocyte proliferative response during the acute infection is significantly greater than that seen in the chronic infection. Typically peripheral blood lymphocytes (PBL) in acute HBV infection will respond to HBV nucleocapsid antigens with a mean stimulation index (measured by ^3H thymidine uptake) of 10.2 (sd 4.5) while that seen in chronic patients is 3.44 (sd 2.28) [11]. Interestingly the mean stimulation index during acute on chronic episodes is 4.39 (sd 1.22) but where the acute episode leads to seroconversion the stimulation index rises to 6.59 (sd 4.58) [12].

These findings suggest two possible strategies of using adoptive transfer to promote viral clearance ; transfer of antigen-specific CTL or transfer of antigen specific $CD4^+$ T helper cells. Currently the use of antigen-specific CTL is being tested in the treatment of post-transplantation CMV infection though no results are yet available [13]. In HBV, however, there is evidence from animal model work that this treatment strategy may work : Chisari and colleagues have administered cloned HBs-specific CTL to HBV-transgenic mice and found that response can be varied by the route of administration and the dose of lymphocytes infused [14]. There is clearly a large gap between these experiments and routinely available immunotherapy and in order to fill this gap we will need to determine to which antigen the response should be directed and the relevant MHC restriction elements for this antigen since autologous CTL will clearly not be available. Moreover clearance of infected hepatocytes alone may not be sufficient to cure the disease as free virus will subsequently re-infect in the absence of neutralising antibody.

The second method of using adoptive transfer as immunotherapy might prove more easily attainable. Expansion of autologous antigen-specific PBL as $CD4^+$ cell lines *in vitro* is a technique which is frequently performed in immunology laboratories. Clones can be generated from these lines and selected clones could be re-infused to promote the $CD4^+$ response *in vivo. In vitro* $CD4^+$ help is essential for supporting CTL formation. Milich's experiments have shown us that anti-HBc antibody formation can occur independently of T cell help but this antibody is present in chronic disease and does not appear to have a role in either viral neutralisation or antibody directed cellular cytotoxicity [15]. The virus neutralising anti-HBs antibody does require $CD4^+$ helper cells, though this may be provided by HBc-specific $CD4^+$ lymphocytes [16]. Consequently adoptive transfer of HBc-specific $CD4^+$ helper cells may augment both the CTL and humoral immune effector machinery of HBV clearance.

Immunotherapy with antibodies

Anti-HBs is a virus neutralising antibody the presence of which confers protection against HBV infection. Interestingly the emergence of this antibody in chronic HBV patients which occurs some months after HBe/anti-HBe sero-conversion is accompanied by loss of serum HBV DNA detectable by PCR [17]. Agammaglobulinaemic patients (with normal cellular immunity) develop an aggressive chronic hepatitis when infected with HBV but are unable to clear the infection through lack of virus neutralising antibody. We have treated two such patients with a murine monoclonal anti-HBs antibody which resulted in clearance of the virus as judged by HBeAg clearance and HBV DNA (dot blot) [18]. Normoglobulinaemic patients could not be treated with this murine antibody due to the formation of anti-species antibodies, so a human antibody has been created by grafting the complementary determining regions.

Absence of the antibody is common to the normoglobulinaemic chronic hepatitis patient as it is to the agammaglobulinaemic. Moreover patients clearing HBsAg following interferon therapy have lower anti-HBs titres than patients who have acute HBV infection [19]. It is therefore proposed to test this antibody in clinical trials involving normoglobulinaemic patients. Hyper-immune anti-HBs globulin is currently used to prevent graft re-infection following transplantation but unfortunately supplies are very expensive and scarce. The humanised monoclonal anti-HBs will soon be submitted to clinical trials in transplant patients and should subsequently eliminate the need for hyperimmune globulin.

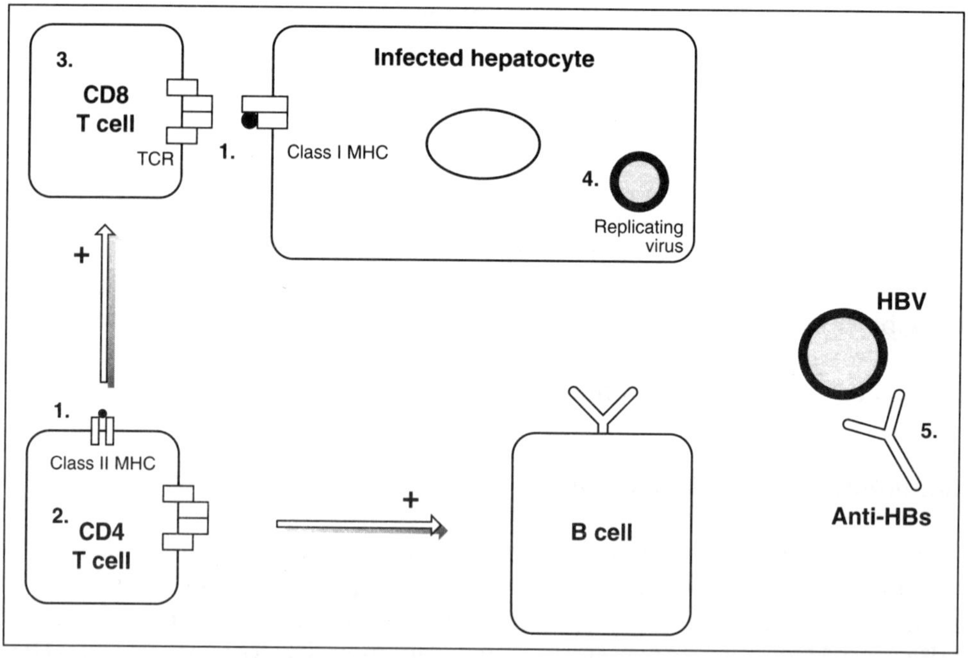

Figure 2. Sites for potential therapeutic intervention in chronic hepatitis B infection. 1. Pharmacological enhancement of antigen presentation. 2. Adoptive transfer of antigen-specific CD4+ T cells. 3. Adoptive transfer of antigen specific CD8+ T cells. 4. Inhibition of viral replication. 5. Administration of recombinant neutralising antibody.

Tailoring therapy

Although the ultimate aim of treatment in patients with chronic HBV infection should be viral clearance, the group of patients is highly heterogeneous and therapy may most efficiently be used by tailoring the therapy to fit the patient.

Agammaglobulinaemics

As has already been discussed, viral persistence in these patients results from their inability to make viral neutralising antibody. Therapy in this minority group should be aimed at surmounting this defect through administration of monoclonal anti-HBs. 10 % to 15 % of normal HBs vaccinees fail to respond with adequate anti-HBs levels and this group can be recognized by a specific MHC haplotype [20]. It is conceivable that a similar proportion of normoglobulinaemic patients are persistently infected for the same reasons and therefore administration of anti-HBs would be appropriate therapy.

Generalised immunosuppression

Although in the majority of patients with chronic HBV infection there is a specific failure of the immune system with respect to HBV, there are groups of patients with a more generalised immune defect, e.g. patients with renal failure and transplantees. In these patients interferon therapy results are poor and other methods of augmenting the HBV specific immune response are unlikely to succeed. In this situation control of viral replication long-term may be the only sensible and attainable goal. It is essential, however, that the therapy chosen should be free of unpleasant side-effects and be available as a simple oral administration. Candidates for this type of treatment are the new dideoxynucleoside analogues and famciclovir as discussed earlier. Short-term clinical trials of these drugs may confirm the ability of the drugs to inhibit replication, but much longer term studies will be needed to demonstrate any effect on prognosis.

Patients with inactive disease

These patients do not respond to interferon therapy and are well represented by the HBV transgenic mouse model where the virus is tolerated by the immune system. Like the transgenic mouse these patients may be susceptible to adoptive transfer of HBV specific CTL. Up to 90 % of hepatocytes may be infected in these patients, so administration of a potent therapy must be carefully controlled to avoid induction of fulminant disease. Again anti-HBs could be used to prevent re-infection of regenerating hepatocytes.

Conclusion

There are many exciting new approaches to the therapy of chronic HBV infection which stem from a better understanding of the pathogenesis of the disease. These may have much to teach us in the parallel fields of management of chronic HCV.

References

1. Thomas HC, Karayiannis P, Brook G. Treatment of hepatitis B virus infection with interferon. Factors predicting response to interferon. J Hepatol 1991 ; 13 (suppl 1) : S4-7.
2. Farraye FA, Mamish DM, Zeldis JB. Preliminary evidence that azidothymidine does not affect hepatitis B virus replication in acquired immunodeficiency syndrome (AIDS) patients. J Med Virol 1989 ; 29 : 266-7.
3. Jacyna MR, Thomas HC. Antiviral therapy : hepatitis B. Br Med Bull 1990 ; 46 : 368-82.
4. Coates JA, Cammack N, Jenkinson HJ, *et al.* The separated enantiomers of 2'-deoxy-3'-thiacytidine (BCH 189) both inhibit human immunodeficiency virus replication *in vitro*. Antimicrob Agents Chemother 1992 ; 36 : 202-5.
5. Galle PR, Theilmann L. Inhibition of hepatitis B virus polymerase-activity by various agents. Transient expression of hepatitis B virus DNA in hepatoma cells as novel system for evaluation of antiviral drugs. Arzneimittelforschung 1990 ; 40 : 1380-2.
6. Freiman JS, Murray SM, Vickery K, Lim D, Cossart YE. Postexposure treatment of experimental DHBV infection : a new therapeutic strategy. J Med Virol 1990 ; 30 : 272-6.
7. Takehara T, Hayashi N, Katayama K, *et al.* Enhanced expression of HLA class I by inhibited replication of hepatitis B virus. J Hepatol 1992 ; 14 : 232-6.
8. Zheng B, Brett S, Tite J, Lifely R, Brodie T, Rhodes J. Galactose oxidation in the design of immunogenic vaccines. Science 1992 ; 256 : 1560-3.
9. Doymaz M, Rouse B. Herpetic stromal keratitis : an immunopathologic disease mediated by CD4+ T lymphocytes. Invest Ophtalmol Vis Sci 1992 ; 33 : 2165-73.
10. Bertoletti A, Ferrari C, Fiaccadori F, *et al.* HLA class I restricted human cytotoxic T cells recognise endogenously synthesized hepatitis B virus nucleocapsid antigen. Proc Natl Acad Sci USA 1991 ; 88 : 10445-9.
11. Ferrari C, Penna A, Bertoletti A, *et al.* Cellular immune response to hepatitis B virus-encoded antigens in acute and chronic hepatitis B virus infection. J Immunol 1990 ; 145 : 3442-9.
12. Tsai S, Chen P, Lai M, *et al.* Acute exacerbations of chronic type B hepatitis are accompanied by increased T cell responses to hepatitis B core and e antigens. J Clin Invest 1992 ; 89 : 87-96.
13. Riddell SR, Reusser P, Greenberg PD. Cytotoxic T cells specific for cytomegalovirus : a potential therapy for immunocompromised patients. Rev Infect Dis 1991 ; 13 (suppl 11) : S966-73.
14. Ando K, Moriyama T, Wirth S, *et al.* Cytotoxic T cell induced fulminant hepatitis in HBV envelope transgenic mice. In : Chisari F, Gowans E, ed. Molecular biology of hepatitis B viruses. La Jolla, California, 1992 : 136.

15. Milich D, McLachlan A. The nucleocapsid of hepatitis B is both a T cell-independent and a T cell-dependent antigen. Science 1986 ; 234 : 1398-401.
16. Milich DR, McLachlan A, Thornton GB, Hughes JL. Antibody production to the nucleocapsid and envelope of the hepatitis B virus primed by a single T cell site. Nature 1987 ; 329 : 547-9.
17. Korenman J, Baker B, Waggoner J, Everhart JE, Di BA, Hoofnagle JH. Long-term remission of chronic hepatitis B after alpha-interferon therapy. Ann Intern Med 1991 ; 114 : 629-34.
18. Lever A, Waters J, Brook M, Karayiannis P, Thomas H. Monoclonal antibody to HBsAg for chronic hepatitis B virus infection with hypogammaglobulinaemia. Lancet 1990 ; 335 : 1529.
19. Karayiannis P, Kanatakis S, Thomas HC. Anti-HBs response in seroconverting chronic HBV carriers following alpha-interferon treatment. J Hepatol 1990 ; 10 : 350-2.
20. Egea E, Iglesias A, Salazar M, *et al.* The cellular basis for lack of antibody response to hepatitis vaccine in humans. J Exp Med 1991 ; 173 : 531-8.
21. Siddiqui A, Gaynor R, Srinivasan A, Mapoles J, Farr RW. Trans-activation of viral enhancers including long-terminal repeat of the human immunodeficiency virus by the hepatitis B virus X protein. Virology 1989 ; 169 : 479-84.
22. Samuel D, Bismuth A, Mathieu D, *et al.* Passive immunoprophylaxis after liver transplantation in HBsAg-positive patients. Lancet 1991 ; 337 : 813-5.

Progress in Hepatology 93. J.P. Miguet and D. Dhumeaux, eds.
John Libbey Eurotext, Paris © 1993, pp. 109-119

12

Hepatitis vaccines : an update

D. SHOUVAL

The Liver Unit, Division of Medicine, Hadassah University Hospital, 91120 Jerusalem, Israel.

Viral hepatitis, regardless of the etiologic agent, is one of the most common infectious diseases worldwide. There is currently no specific treatment for established acute hepatitis A, B, C, D, or E, and antiviral treatment of chronic hepatitis B or C has met with limited success. It seems that on a global basis, prevention of viral hepatitis would be a much more achievable goal, as compared to treatment of established infection(s) and the long-term complications. Indeed, the past twelve years have been very rewarding as to the development and clinical evaluation of vaccines against hepatitis B virus (HBV), and, recently, hepatitis A virus (HAV) infections. Attempts at developing experimental vaccines against hepatitis C, D and E virus infections are in progress. Therefore, the clinical hepatologist today must be aware of the various prevention strategies against viral hepatitis in order to offer his/her patients at risk the best available protection. The following pages will provide the reader with a brief update on many of the recent developments in prevention of HAV and HVB infections.

Vaccines against hepatitis A virus infection

The recent progress in development of new vaccines against HAV infection requires an examination of the epidemiology, the tools to evaluate efficacy, and the rationale for introduction of another new vaccine into clinical practice.

Epidemiology and clinical course

HAV infection has been known for thousands of years. Its major route of transmission is through fecal-oral contamination or intake of contaminated water or food, but transmission through blood products may rarely occur. Compared to infection with other hepatitis viruses, the outcome of HAV infection is usually favorable, although the disease can cause significant morbidity in adolescents and adults, as shown in the recent Shanghai epidemic [1]. On rare occasions, it may lead to fulminant liver failure associated with a 40 % mortality rate unless liver transplantation is attempted. Occasionally 3 % to 20 % of individuals may develop a relapsing form of HAV, or a protracted course which may take months to resolve [2]. The changing prevalence of HAV infection worldwide, which is the outcome of improved socio-economic and sanitary conditions, has led to a decline in infection rates and to a shift towards infection at an older age as compared to 20 and 40 years ago. Therefore, adult populations, mainly in the developed countries, but also in former developing countries, are susceptible to HAV infection which is more symptomatic and incapacitating as compared to the frequently asymptomatic course in young children.

Diagnosis of HAV infection and monitoring of immune response to vaccination

HAV belongs to the picornavirus family (genus Hep A-RNA) and contains a single stranded 7.48 kb linear positive-sense RNA. Four major HAV genotypes have been identified in humans from different geographic location, with a nucleotide sequence variability of 15 % to 25 % in the VP_1 region [3]. Four polypeptides, VP_1-VP_4, are cleaved from a precursor polyprotein, but only one serotype is known. The non-enveloped HAV is extremely resistant to heat, ether, and disinfectants. Wild type HAV is difficult to grow in tissue culture, and continuous propagation in culture has been associated with development of several mutations which do not affect the conventional serologic markers for infection. Until recently, infection in experimental animals and in humans was monitored through immunological assays based on detection of immunoglobulin M or G to the capsid proteins. These conventional assays have an excellent record for diagnosis of HAV infection and immunity after « natural » infection, but have limitations with regard to monitoring the humoral immune response following passive immunization with immune serum globulin (Ig) or after active vaccination. The recently established modified HAVAB assay [4] may increase the sensitivity of the conventional HAVAB (Abbott, N. Chicago, IL) assay by using a 10-fold higher serum test sample (100 μl instead of 10 μl) ; thus, threshold of detection can be reduced from 100 to 10mlU/ml. Using the modified HAVAB assay, antibodies to HAV (anti-HAV, total) may be detected in recipients of Ig or inactivated hepatitis A vaccines (iHAV) [5]. Other immunoassays, such as the enzyme-linked assay developed by Smith Kline Biologicals (SKB) have also been used to monitor post-vaccination anti-HAV [6]. Unfortunately, no data are available as yet which compare sensitivity and specificity of the modified HAVAB assay to the SKB ELISA, and standardization of assays is necessary for better assessment of the comparative immunogenicity of the newly developed HAV vaccines. The heterogeneity of the currently available solid phase competitive inhibition immunoassays for detection of anti-HAV is manifested by a variable capacity of these assays to detect low and high affinity antibodies to HAV. Antibody response to HAV vaccines may be measured by a number of more accurate techniques, which are, however, more complicated, time-consuming, and costly, and are currently used only in research laboratories. These assays, which are designed to detect neutralizing antibodies to HAV, include the radio immuno focus inhibition test (RIFIT), the hepatitis A virus antigen reduction assay (HAVARNA), and a new radioimmunoprecipitation assay [7]. The immunoprecipitation assay seems so far to be the most sensitive and technically useful assay of the three techniques listed. Virus neutralization assays for detection of neutralizing antibodies are significantly more sensitive than competitive inhibition assays, although they are less standardized and significantly more time consuming and laborious. Other research tools for monitoring HAV infection include experimental assays to distinguish between the immune response in acquired HAV infection and response to vaccine through the monitoring of antibodies to non-structural proteins from the P_2 and P_3 regions of the HAV genome (not present in vaccinees), detection of HAV antigen in stool or culture, and detection of HAV RNA in serum by conventional hybridization or by RT-PCR.

Passive immunization with immune serum globulin (Ig)

For the past 40 years, and until recently, Ig produced from human plasma pools manufactured by alcohol fractionation for i.m. injection has been the only available means for short-term or post-exposure prophylaxis against hepatitis A. The two recommended doses (0.02 ml/kg and 0.06 ml/kg) will provide protection against clinical hepatitis A for 4 to 6 months. Despite its excellent safety and efficacy record, administration of Ig has several limitations. These include : the necessity for repeated immunization for longer protection, which is accompanied by inconvenience, discomfort, and increased cost ; the unknown hazards of potentially harmful agents produced from pools of human serum ; the interference with diagnostic tests for other etiologic agents, such as HIV ; or interference with vaccination efficacy, such as against measles, mumps, and rubella. In some countries, populations at risk may receive repeated injections of Ig for many years, while the effect of repeated immunization with human serum proteins remains unknown. Finally, the worldwide decline in prevalence of anti-HAV has led to the dwindling of anti-HAV titers in pooled serum used for preparation of Ig. Thus protection of large populations, such as military personnel during the Gulf War, or civilian populations during the Shanghai epidemic, became more difficult. Administration of Ig at 0.06 ml/kg leads to immediate protection against clinical hepatitis A, with anti-HAV titers reaching approximately 60 to 100 mlU/ml, and sufficient levels of neutralizing antibodies as early as 48 hours after injection. Generally, following Ig injection, anti-HAV levels will fall rapidly to become undetectable, or below protective levels, within 8 to 16 weeks. However, protection may last for 6 to 9 months following a single injection, even when anti-HAV is undetectable by the methods currently in use.

Active immunization against HAV

Propagation of HAV in culture has led to development of both a live attenuated candidate vaccine, as well as several formalin inactivated alum adjuvanted vaccines derived from attenuated strains adapted for growth in culture [5, 6, 8-13]. A live attenuated vaccine has been tested in a small number of volunteers and found to be immunogenic when administered by injection [8]. However, in the past four years, most efforts have been concentrated on evaluation of the safety, tolerability, immunogenicity, and protective efficacy of formalin inactivated (« killed ») HAV vaccines (iHAV) [5, 8-13]. Two of these vaccines, namely HAVRIX™ [6, 10] and VAQTA™ [5, 11], produced by SKB and Merck & Co., respectively, have already been administered to many thousands of adults and children worldwide. Both vaccines were found to be highly immunogenic and very well tolerated, leading to 100 % seroconversion ($\geqslant$ 10 mlU/ml of anti-HAV) in children and young adults, following one or two injections. Two immunization strategies are now being tested : administration of two doses given at 0 and 6 months, or three doses given at 0, 1, and 6 months. The available data suggest that > 90 % of young vaccinees will seroconvert within 19 to 30 days of a single dose injection. Attempts are now being made to increase seroconversion rates in the first 2 to 4 weeks following primary immunization with 25 to 50 units of the VAQTA™, or with 720-1440 ELISA units of HAVRIX™. To date, no comparative controlled data are available yet on the antigen content and quantitative anti-HAV response in vaccinees receiving VAQTA™ or HAVRIX™.

Nevertheless, both vaccines seem to lead to unprecedented seroconversion rates. Both vaccines have been shown to protect chimpanzees or marmosets against challenge with wild type HAV. Protective efficacy trials have been initiated for HAVRIX™ in Thailand and Chile [10, 14], and for VAQTA™ in Monroe, New York [15]. In Thailand, in a randomized trial, 40,119 children received either iHAV or a recombinant hepatitis B vaccine. Study design in Thailand has so far enabled the evaluation of protective efficacy of HAVRIX™ after 2 or 3 doses of 360 ELISA units, given at 0, 1, and 6 months. There were 29 cases of acute HAV infection in a representative sample of placebo recipients, and only 1 case among iHAV recipients, thus establishing the protective efficacy after 2 doses for HAVRIX™ [14]. A different immunization strategy was used to study the protective efficacy of VAQTA™, in a placebo-controlled trial conducted in 1,037 children, aged from 2 to 16 years, in Monroe, New York [15]. The Monroe study design was based on the hypothesis that a single 25 unit dose would lead to 100 % seroconversion in young adults [5]. In this study, children received two doses of iHAV, administered at 0 and at 6, 12, or 18 months. Data available following injection of the first 25 units doses of VAQTA™ indicated that 25 out of 518 children receiving placebo injection, and none of the 519 children receiving iHAV, developed clinical hepatitis A virus infection between 19 to 50 days after a single dose immunization.

These results suggest at 100 % protective efficacy for VAQTA™ in children and adolescents. The iHAV vaccine tested was extremely well tolerated, and established the efficacy of the new vaccine which, in fact, led to a rapid cessation of a serious HAV outbreak in this community. Experimental evidence to date indicates that seroconversion after a single iHAV injection confers immune memory which will respond to a booster dose given at 6 months, with a rapid anamnestic response. Available data also suggest that protection against clinical HAV infection may last 5 to 10 years. Many issues concerning the strategy of immunization and biologic properties of iHAV vaccines remain open, and will be addressed in the next 1 to 2 years. These include definition of target populations for immunization (i.e. travellers, day care and nursery workers, food handlers, and military personnel). Furthermore, the precise minimal interval between primary immunization and inception of protection against clinical hepatitis A is still not established. In children there is convincing evidence that protection begins at least 3 weeks after the first dose. It is essential to shorten this interval in order to be able to provide quicker post, or even pre, exposure prophylaxis. Other factors that may affect this interval include weight, age, and sex of vaccinee. Studies are now in progress to address these issues. It is hoped that by increasing the dose of iHAV and/or the amount of adjuvant, the period required to induce seroconversion may be shortened. Meanwhile, induction of immediate protection against clinical HAV infection may require passive/active immunization with simultaneous administration of Ig and iHAV. Preliminary data suggest that concurrent administration of both compounds is well tolerated and leads to a rapid rise in anti-HAV levels, although at a marginally lower level as compared to iHAV alone. Currently, the formalin inactivated hepatitis A vaccine, HAVRIX™, is already licensed in a few European countries [10], and soon, both iHAV vaccines are expected to be available in many Western countries. Second generation recombinant vaccines have so far failed to induce neutralizing antibodies to HAV, although this approach is still being tested. It is expected that within a few years, results of clinical trials using combination vaccines against HAV, HBV, and DTP will have a major impact on immunization policies worldwide.

Vaccines against hepatitis B virus infection

Active immunization against HBV infection is now common practice [16-19]. Initially, plasma derived vaccines (PDV), containing purified hepatitis B virus surface antigen(s) (HBsAg), received only partial acceptance. Second generation, yeast derived vaccines (YDV) against HBV are now in use worldwide. Both plasma and yeast derived vaccines have had an excellent safety record, with rare exceptions [20-26]. To date, the rationale for universal immunization of neonates against HBV in countries with high or intermediate endemicity of HBV is widely accepted [18]. Indeed, over 40 countries are in the process of introducing universal immunization into their EPI program, or have already done so. Cost is the major limiting factor affecting implementation of universal immunization to neonates in Africa and most Asian countries. Data obtained through cost-benefit analysis in the past decade repeatedly suggest a long-term benefit of such an immunization policy [27, 28]. However, many countries are unable to allocate the short-term funds necessary to introduce an effective prevention program against HBV, even though the long-term cost-benefit analysis justifies such an effort.

Advocates of worlwide immunization programs have revived the use of the relatively low cost PDV in several countries in East Asia. Dwindling of the plasma pools from HBsAg carriers required for preparation of PDVs will eventually lead to increased demand for YDV. Indeed, large scale production of non-glycosylated HBsAg in yeasts is already cost effective, and costs are declining rapidly [18]. The available HBV vaccines, whether PDV or YDV, are highly immunogenic, leading to 90 % to 96 % seroconversion rates in pediatric and young adult populations. However, 4 % to 10 % of vaccine recipients are non-responders or low responders. Furthermore, there are a number of target populations which do not readily seroconvert when immunized with the conventional HBV vaccines. These groups include immunosuppressed patients, chronic dialysis patients, and older adults. Finally, several escape mutants of HBV have recently been described, which emerged in association with active immunization using HBsAg alone [29, 30]. Therefore, there is a limited rationale for developing more immunogenic vaccines. The present update will concentrate on the recent development of third generation recombinant vaccines against HBV.

New third-generation hepatitis B vaccines

Native HBV surface particles contain three different compounds : the small HBs protein in a non-glycosylated (P24) and glycosylated (GP27) form ; the middle HBs protein (P33 and GP36) ; and the large HBs protein (P39 and GP42). The small (SHBs), middle (MHBs), and large (LHBs) HBs proteins were formerly termed S, pre S_2 and pre S_1 antigens, respectively [31]. The two additional LHBs and MHBs domains seem to play a major role in attachment of HBV to hepatocytes. Furthermore, antibodies against these antigens have been shown independently to be protective against experimental challenge of chimpanzees against HBV, and sequential domains of these pre S proteins may play a role in generation of T helper cell dependent anti-HBs response. During the past 4 or 5 years, attempts have been made to develop more immunogenic HBV vaccines containing, in addition to the S antigen, one or both of the pre S proteins. Initially, pre S_2 and pre S_1 antigens were expressed in yeasts. Experimental yeast derived vaccines, containing either pre S_2 alone or pre S_2 and pre S_1 antigens, seemed originally to be more immunogenic as compared to SHBs (S) containing vaccines. However, initial higher seroconversion rates and higher anti-HBs titers observed in pilot studies conducted in experimental animals and humans were not reproduced in larger scale studies.

Thus, attempts to produce a more immunogenic yeast derived vaccine with proper conformation of all three surface proteins have not yet met with full success. However, it is still possible that inclusion of sequential epitopes of pre S_1 in HBV vaccines designed to induce a helper T cell response will improve its immunogenicity. Investigators in France, Israel, Japan, China, and Germany have independently explored an alternative expression system for HBV surface proteins using the mammalian derived Chinese hamster ovary (CHO) cell line [31-38]. To date, experimental lots of CHO derived vaccines containing glycosylated and non-glycosylated S and pre S_2 proteins have been tested in mice and humans [32, 36]. Preliminary data suggest a markedly enhanced anti-HBs response and a lower rate of non- or hypo-responders. However, attempts at upscaling production with one vaccine prototype resulted in less immunogenic vaccine lots, suggesting also a stability problem. Controlled randomized clinical trials comparing these new vaccines with the conventional vaccines tested in the special groups of non-responders, including also immunosuppressed and dialysis patients, are still not completed.

Recently, a new CHO derived vaccine, which expresses mainly the S protein, but also small amounts of pre S_2 and pre S_1 (glycosylated and non-glycosylated) has been shown to be much more immunogenic in mice and in small scale studies in humans, as compared to yeast derived S vaccines [33, 35, 38]. In these preliminary studies, genetically restricted resistance to the S antigen in special strains of mice was shown to be abolished through vaccination with the S - pre S_2 - pre S_1, CHO derived vaccine [35]. However, analysis of data on immunogenicity of new HBV vaccines in mice requires caution, since immunogenicity in humans may not necessarily be the same. Nevertheless, unpublished data on children immunized with CHO derived HBV vaccines at HBsAg doses ranging from 2.5 to 10 μg indicate that approximately 25 % of vaccinees developed anti-HBs titers of between 10^4 and 10^6 mIU/ml, a level which exceeds by far the titers obtained after immunization with yeast derived non- glycosylated S particles. The reason for this augmented immunogenicity of the CHO derived vaccines is not completely understood. Different physical properties of the CHO derived S particles which are secreted into the growth medium may also contribute to the enhanced immunogenicity irrespective of the co-expression of pre S_1 and/or pre S_2 epitopes. Preliminary cost-benefit analysis indicates that production of CHO derived vaccine is more costly as compared to the yeast derived vaccine. Therefore, there will be a limited justification for the use of CHO derived vaccines in special risk groups, such as non-responders, immunosuppressed patients, patients on dialysis, and older adults. These third-generation experimental vaccines will be judged mainly based on their potential property of inducing higher seroconversion rates, but not necessarily the higher anti-HBs titers. Finally, development of such vaccines which may lead to enhanced immunogenicity should by no means affect the continually increasing distribution of the conventional vaccines for prevention of HBV worldwide.

*

* *

In conclusion, a number of recently developed vaccines against hepatitis A and B virus infections are currently undergoing clinical trials. Two formalin inactivated vaccines against hepatitis A virus (HAV) infection have been prepared from inactivated (killed) attenuated HAV strains propagated in tissue culture. In two protective efficacy trials conducted in Thailand and in the USA, one or two doses of these HAV vaccines were shown to effectively protect children and adolescents against clinical hepatitis A. Experimental vaccines against hepatitis B virus (HBV) infection, containing S, pre S_2, and pre S_1 antigens, have been prepared in yeasts and Chinese hamster ovary cells. Early studies with some of these vaccines indicated an enhanced immunogenicity as compared with conventional plasma or yeast derived vaccines containing only the non-glycosylated small surface protein.

References

1. Xu ZY, Li ZH, Wang JX, Xiao ZP, Dong DX. Ecology and prevention of a shellfish-associated hepatitis A epidemic in Shanghai, China. Vaccine 1992 ; 10 : S67-8.
2. Glikson M, Galun E, Oren R, Tur-Kaspa R, Shouval D. Relapsing hepatitis A : review of 14 cases and literature survey. Medicine 1992 ; 71 : 14-23.
3. Lemon SM, Jansen RW, Brown EA. Genetic antigenic differences between strains of hepatitis A virus. Vaccine 1992 ; 10 : S40-4.
4. Provost PJ, Bishop RP, Gerety RJ, *et al.* New findings in live attenuated hepatitis A vaccine development. J Med Virol 1986 ; 20 : 165-75.
5. Shouval D, Ashur Y, Adler R, *et al.* Single and booster dose responses to an inactivated hepatitis A virus vaccine : comparison with immune serum globulin prophylaxis. Vaccine 1993 ; 11 : S9-14.
6. André FE, D'Hondt E, Delern A, Safary A. Clinical assessment of the safety and efficacy of an inactivated hepatitis A vaccine : rationale and summary of findings. Vaccine 1992 ; 10 : S160-8.
7. Lemon SM. Inactivated hepatitis A virus vaccines (Editorial). Hepatology 1992 ; 15 : 1194-7.

8. Midthun K, Ellerbeck E, Gershman K, *et al.* Safety and immunogenicity of a live attenuated hepatitis A virus vaccine in seronegative volunteers. J Infect Dis 1991 ; 163 : 735-9.
9. Siegl G, Lemon SM. Recent advances in hepatitis A vaccine development. Virus Res 1990 ; 17 : 55-92.
10. Hollinger B, André FA, Melnick J, eds. Proceedings of the International Symposium on Active Immunization Against Hepatitis A. Vaccine 1992 ; 10 : S1-174.
11. Shouval D, ed. Proceedings of an International Satellite Symposium on Active Immunization Against Hepatitis A. J Hepatol 1993 (Supplement), in press.
12. Flehmig B, Heinricy U, Pfisterer M. Immunogenicity of a killed hepatitis A vaccine in seronegative volunteers. Lancet 1989 ; 1 : 1039-41.
13. Sjögren MH, Hoke CH, Binn LN, *et al.* Immunogenicity of an inactivated hepatitis A vaccine. Ann Intern Med 1991 ; 114 : 470-1.
14. Innis BL, Snitbhan R, Kunasol P, *et al.* Field efficacy trial of inactivated hepatitis A vaccine among children in Thailand (an extended abstract). Vaccine 1992 ; 10 : S159.
15. Werzberg A, Mensch B, Kuter B, *et al.* A controlled trial of a formalin-inactivated hepatitis A vaccine in healthy children. N Engl J Med 1992 ; 327 : 453-7.
16. Hepatitis B virus : a comprehensive strategy for eliminating transmission in the US through universal childhood vaccination. Recommendations of the Immunization Practices Advisory Committee (ACIP). Morbid Mortal Week Rep 1991 ; 22, 13 : 1-25.
17. Hadler SC, Margolis HS. Hepatitis B immunization : vaccine types, efficacy and indications for immunization. Curr Clin Top Infect Dis 1992 ; 12 : 282-308.
18. Proceedings of the International Conference on Prospects for Eradication of Hepatitis B Virus. Blumberg BS, Hepburn A, André FE, eds. Vaccine 1990 ; 8 : S1-139.
19. Committee on Infectious Disease, American Academy of Pediatrics. Universal hepatitis B immunization, Pediatrics 1992 ; 89 : 795-800.
20. Shaw FF, Graham DJ, Guess HA, *et al.* Post marketing surveillance for neurologic adverse events reported after hepatitis B vaccination. Experience with the first three years. Am J Epidemiol 1988 ; 127 : 337-52.
21. Hudson TJ, Newkirk M, Gervais F, Shuster J. Adverse reactions to the recombinant hepatitis B vaccine. J Allergy Clin Immunol 1991 ; 88 : 821-2.
22. McMahon BJ, Helminiak C, Wainwright RB, Bulkow L, Trimble BA, Wainwright K. Frequency of adverse reactions to hepatitis B vaccine in 43,618 persons. Am J Med 1992 ; 92 : 254-6.
23. Duclos P. Adverse events after hepatitis B vaccination. Can Med Assoc J 1992 ; 147 : 1023-6.
24. Wakeel RA, White MI. Erythema multiforme associated with hepatitis B vaccine. Br J Dermatol 1992 ; 126 : 94-5 (letter).
25. Herroelen L, de Keyser J, Ebinger G. Central nervous system demyelination after immunization with recombinant hepatitis B vaccine. Lancet 1991 ; 338 : 1174-5.
26. O'Sullivan SJ. Alleged link between hepatitis B vaccine and chronic fatigue syndrome. Can Med Assoc J 1992 ; 15 : 399-402.
27. Arevalo JA, Washington E. Cost effectiveness of prenatal screening and immunization for hepatitis B virus. JAMA 1988 ; 259 : 365-9.
28. Ginsberg GM, Shouval D. Cost-benefit analysis of a nationwide inoculation programme against hepatitis in an area of intermediate endemicity. J Epidemiol Community Health 1992 ; 46 : 587-94.
29. Harrison TJ, Hopes EA, Oon CJ, Zanetti AR, Zuckerman AJ. Independent emergence of a vaccine induced escape mutant of hepatitis B virus. J Hepatol 1991 ; 4 : S105-7.
30. Okamoto H, Yano K, Nozaki Y, *et al.* Mutations within the S gene of hepatitis B virus transmitted from mothers to babies immunized with hepatitis B immune globulin and vaccine. Pediatr Res 1992 ; 32 : 264-8.
31. Gerlich WH, Deepen R, Heermann KH, *et al.* Protective potential of hepatitis B virus antigens other than the S gene protein. Vaccine 1990 ; 8 : S63-8.
32. Coursaget P, Bringer L, Sarv G, *et al.* Comparative immunogenicity in children of mammalian cell derived recombinant hepatitis B vaccine and plasma derived hepatitis B vaccine. Vaccine 1992 ; 10 : 379-82.

33. Yap I, Guan R, Chan SH. Comparison of immunogenicity of a pre-S containing HBV vaccine with non-preS-containing vaccines. In : Nishioka K, ed. Proceedings of the International Symposium on Viral Hepatitis and Liver Disease, 8th Triennial Congress, Tokyo, Viral Hepatitis Research Foundation of Japan 1993 ; 86 (abstract).
34. Hemmerling AE, Müller R, Firusian N, Haubitz M, Thoma HA. Clinical experience with the pre-S1 containing vaccine (HG-3) in different non-responder groups. In : Nishioka K, ed. Proceedings of the International Symposium on Viral Hepatitis and Liver Disease, 8th Triennial Congress, Tokyo, Viral Hepatitis Research Foundation of Japan 1993 ; 86 (abstract).
35. Shouval D, Ilan Y, Hourvitz A, *et al.* Immunogenicity of a recombinant hepatitis B vaccine containing pre S_1 and pre S_2 antigens in mice and humans. In : Nishioka K, ed. Proceedings of the International Symposium on Viral Hepatitis and Liver Disease, 8th Triennial Congress, Tokyo, Viral Hepatitis Research Foundation of Japan 1993 ; 87 (abstract).
36. Akahane Y. Clinical trial of a preS_2-containing hepatitis B vaccine : early response of anti-pre S_2 in vaccinees and efficacy in non-responders to conventional vaccines. In : Nishioka K, ed. Proceedings of the International Symposium on Viral Hepatitis and Liver Disease, 8th Triennial Congress, Tokyo, Viral Hepatitis Research Foundation of Japan 1993 ; 48 (abstract).
37. Yao FL. An efficacy trial of a mammalian cell derived recombinant DNA hepatitis B vaccine in infants born to mothers positive for HBsAg in Shangai, China. Int J Epidemiol 1991 ; 21 : 564-73.
38. Yap I, Guan R, Chan SH. Recombinant DNA hepatitis B vaccine containing pre-S components of the HBV coat protein — a preliminary study on immunogenicity. Vaccine 1992 ; 10 : 439-42.

Progress in Hepatology 93. J.P. Miguet and D. Dhumeaux, eds.
John Libbey Eurotext, Paris © 1993, pp. 121-125

13

Hepatitis delta infection and liver transplantation

M. RIZZETTO[1], A. OTTOBRELLI[2], A. SMEDILE[2]

[1] *Institute of Internal Medicine, University of Turin, Italy.*
[2] *Division of Gastroenterology, Molinette Hospital , Turin, Italy.*

Because the hepatitis delta virus (HDV) requires for *in vivo* infection obligatory helper functions from the hepatitis B virus (HBV), hepatitis D can occur only in individuals who carry the hepatitis B surface antigen in blood. The prevalence of HDV infection is low in the total HBsAg-positive population but sharply increases in HBV carriers who have liver disease, with the highest rates at the two clinical extremes of acute and chronic liver disease, i.e. in carriers with fulminant or cirrhotic liver failure. An ominous feature of HDV disease is also the tendency to more rapidly progress than either hepatitis B or hepatitis C, thus evolving to cirrhosis at earlier ages than the other types of viral hepatitis. These characteristics explain why HDV segregates among HBsAg carriers who are candidates to liver transplantation, despite its negligible prevalence in the general HBsAg-positive population.

While liver transplantation has established an impressive record of cure in all forms of terminal liver diseases, patients transplanted for viral infections of the liver stand a high risk of reinfection and recurrence of the original disease in the graft. The risk is high in patients with ordinary HBV infections ; it is prohibitive in those with viremia detectable by conventional hybridization assays, yet less consistent in patients without HBV viremia. In theory, patients with HDV disease should be at the lowest risk of reinfection, as in the course of chronic hepatitis D HDV inhibits the replication of HBV to such an extent that HBV replication markers are usually not detectable in the blood of these patients. The corollary of these viral interactions to liver transplantation is that the failure to transmit HBV to the graft should also prevent transmission of HDV.

The transplant reality, however, has confirmed only in part these optimistic premises ; more intriguing, it has raised a number of unexpected issues that are changing our views on the pathobiology of hepatitis D and on the interactions between HDV and its helper virus.

Liver transplantation in HDV hepatitis

Patients

We consider in this review a total of 57 HDV transplants reported in three studies [1-3] for whom an adequate follow-up was available.

Twenty-seven patients (group 1) were transplanted in Torino, Milano (Osp. Maggiore) and Bruxelles (UCL). Fifteen patients (group 2) were transplanted in Milano (Osp. Niguarda). Fifteen patients (group 3) were transplanted in Villejuif, France. Only six of the twenty-seven patients in group 1 were given long-term prophylaxis with hyperimmune anti-HBs immunoglobulins (HBIg) whereas eight of the fifteen patients in group 2 and all the patients in group 3 received protection with anti-HBs.

Clinical and virologic post-transplant course

Of the twenty-seven patients in group 1 seven were not reinfected with either HBV and HDV. Twenty became reinfected. Thirteen were reinfected with HDV alone ; this reinfection was precocious, occurring a few days to a few weeks after transplantation. Seven patients became simultaneously reinfected with HDV and HBV several months after transplantation. Overall twelve patients developed a recurrence of hepatitis D ; they included the seven patients reinfected simultaneously with HBV and HDV and five of the thirteen patients originally reinfected by HDV alone ; these five patients remained well and symptom-free while harbouring HDV alone but experienced hepatitis when HBV returned to the graft a few months after HDV reinfection. The eight patients with persistent HDV infection not accompanied by HBV infection are well and symptom-free after follow-up periods varying from 12 to 48 months ; HDV-RNA remains detectable in all (in a few after amplification with the polymerase chain reaction).

HBV/HDV reinfection occurred in four of the seven patients in group 2 who were not given HBIg ; in one such patient HDV recurred 10 days after transplantation followed by recurrence of HBV several weeks later. Remarkably, none of the seven patients in this group who were given HBIg had a viral recurrence.

HDV infection recurred in each of the fifteen patients in group 3, all of whom were protected with HBIg. In seven of these patients HDV returned together with HBV, while in a further patient the return of HDV was followed by the recurrence of HBV several weeks later. Of the seven patients with isolated HDV infection, six lost HDV after 2 years and the seventh lost the virus during the third year of follow-up. All the patients with double HBV/HDV reinfection had liver disease ; one such patient, however, experienced hepatitis as late as 4 years after transplantation.

Histologic course

In three of the twenty-four patients who had double HBV/HDV infections and developed recurrent hepatitis, the disease ran an acute self-limited course followed by resolution of HBV and HDV reinfection [2] ; in the others, infection and hepatitis progressed to chronicity. The histologic follow-up, available from thirteen patients with chronic hepatitis D, has shown progression to cirrhosis in ten and the persistence of minimal hepatic lesions in the other three. No patient has died of recurrent liver disease in the interim.

Discussion

Contrary to the belief that HDV can be spread only under circumstances that transmit also HBV, the model of liver transplantation has shown that the « defective virus » can be transmitted independently from HBV. These « autonomous » HDV infections are harmless and the patients remain symptom-free unless HBV recurs in the liver graft. Upon reactivation of HBV, synthesis of HDV increases (with spreading of the HD-Ag in liver and release of virions to the blood) and HDV infection becomes pathogenic : all HBV/HDV reinfected patients experienced hepatitis, with two French cases developing disease as late as 1 to 4 years after the recurrence of HBV.

HDV-reinfected transplants who were not reinfected with HBV have remained well. In these subjects the fate of viremia is controversial, as in the French series they all lost HDV RNA over the long-term, while viremia is still detectable in all the Italian patients.

In transplants who developed recurrent hepatitis D, the disease has often been rapidly evolutive with ten or thirteen patients progressing to cirrhosis in a matter of 1 to 3 years.

Detailed histological analysis of liver biopsies obtained from nine patients at the onset of recurrent hepatitis D has shown two types of liver lesions [4]. In four patients, the rise of ALT corresponded to necroinflammation, as in typical viral hepatitis and HBV recurred in the form of a productive infection, with the expression of the full battery of HBV markers (including the HBcAg in the liver). In the other five patients, the histological aspects which corresponded to a clinical picture of acute hepatitis (ALT > 15 the upper normal value, jaundice) were degenerative lesions consisting of ballooning degeneration, micro- and macrosteatosis, and eosinophilic alterations of the cytoplasms ; inflammation was absent and the pattern of HBV reinfection was unusual, featuring the HBsAg in blood but lacking HBcAg in the liver.

The latter histologic pattern is apparently related to activation of HDV triggered by an incomplete, atypical HBV infection (as it is often the case in patients with hepatitis D) and appears to be peculiar to HDV infection among viral infection in temperate climates ; however, it is not unique to the transplantation model, as a steatotic vacuolization of the liver cytoplasm has distinguished also severe forms of HDV liver disorders in Indians living in the Amazon Basin [5].

The development of atypical infection profiles explains why only a minority of HDV transplants suffered from hepatitis recurrence despite a high-rate of reinfection. Many of the patients became reinfected with HDV, yet HBV did not recur, thus failing to activate HDV to disease expression ; although HBIg was ineffective in preventing the recurrence of HDV, in most cases it was nevertheless efficacious in preventing reactivation of HBV and the relapse of disease.

*
* *

In conclusion, liver transplantation has a very consistent curative rate in HDV transplants, despite a high risk of reinfection with HDV. HBIg is efficacious in preventing hepatitis D relapse as long as it prevents recurrence of HBV.

However, in the unfortunate minority of patients who have a relapse of hepatitis D, the disease is often progressive, advancing rapidly to cirrhosis with a timing similar to that seen in recurrent hepatitis B.

The liver transplantation model has suggested that HDV can establish latent, non-pathogenic infections, that activation of these infections to disease depends on HBV reactivation and that the histologic pattern of hepatitis D may be modulated by the type of HBV reinfection. Further transmission studies have been designed and executed in the mouse in order to prove these hypotheses. Preliminary results [6] appear to confirm that HDV can be transmitted without « live » HBV in this animal. If this were also the case in humans, HDV might exist in healthy subjects who lack HBsAg and might convert into a pathogen only upon HBV superinfection.

References

1. Ottobrelli A, Marzano A, Smedile A, *et al.* Patterns of hepatitis delta virus reinfection and disease in liver transplantation. Gastroenterology 1991 ; 101 : 1649-55.
2. Bettale G, Alberti A, Saverio L, *et al.* Recurrence of HDV infection after liver transplantation. In : Hepatitis delta virus : molecular biology, pathogenesis and clinical aspects. New York : Wiley-Liss Inc., 1993 : 403-7.
3. Zignego AL, Samuel D, Gigou M, *et al.* Patterns of hepatitis delta reinfection after liver transplantation and their evolution during a long-term follow-up. In : Hepatitis delta virus : molecular biology, pathogenesis and clinical aspects. New York : Wiley-Liss Inc., 1993 ; 409-17.
4. David E, Rahier J, Pucci A, *et al.* Recurrence of hepatitis D (delta) in liver transplants : histopathological aspects. Gastroenterology 1993 ; 104 : 1122-8.
5. Popper H, Thung SN, Gerber MA, *et al.* Histologic studies of severe delta agent infection in Venezuelan Indians. Hepatology 1983 ; 3 : 906-12.
6. Netter HJ, Kajino K, Tailor J. Replication of HDV in the mouse. In : Hepatitis delta virus : molecular biology, pathogenesis and clinical aspects. New York : Wiley-Liss Inc., 1993 : 171-3.

is efficacious in preventing hepatitis D relapse as long as it prevents recurrence of HBV.

However, in the unfortunate minority of patients who have a relapse of hepatitis D, the disease is often progressive, mimicking [illegible] to [illegible] with a [illegible] similar to that seen in recurrent hepatitis B.

[illegible]

Progress in Hepatology 93. J.P. Miguet and D. Dhumeaux, eds.
John Libbey Eurotext, Paris © 1993, pp. 127-133

14

Biliary tract complications following liver transplantation

K. BOUDJEMA, D. JAECK, P. WOLF, J. CINQUALBRE

Centre de Chirurgie Viscérale et de Transplantation, Hôpital de Hautepierre, 67098 Strasbourg Cedex, France.

Biliary tract complications after orthotopic liver transplantation (OLT) are serious events that still take place in 7 % to 30 % of the large series [1-3]. They are usually described as melting pots, full of leaks, necrosis, obstructions or strictures, affecting all or part of the intra-or extrahepatic biliary tract, and occur at different rates depending on the technique that has been used for biliary reconstruction.

Based upon our own experience of 286 liver transplants performed between January 1986 and December 1992, and upon the results reported in the literature, this report attempts to rationally classify the biliary complications which occur after OLT, in order to suggest a logical strategy for both diagnosis and treatment.

Methods of bile duct reconstruction

Up to now, two major techniques of biliary reconstruction have been used : when the recipient common duct is anatomically preserved, the acceptable technique of biliary reconstruction is an end-to-end anastomosis between the donor and recipient common ducts (choledochocholedochostomy) [4]. This anastomosis is generally stented and drained with a T tube that is inserted through a small incision in the recipient bile duct at 10 to 15 mm from the anastomosis. But when the recipient bile duct is not available or is abnormal (biliary atresia, cholangiocarcinoma, alveolar echinococcosis, sclerosing cholangitis), the second technique, consisting of an end-to-side choledocho-jejunostomy, has to be performed, using a 50 to 60-cm defunctionalized jejunum limb.

Various types of biliary complications

Irrespective of the technique used to restore the biliary tract, biliary complications following OLT can be separated into four groups.

Biliary reconstruction complications are the most frequent. They include complications that occur on the extrahepatic biliary tract. The intrahepatic biliary tract is not affected and the hepatic artery is patent.

Anastomotic complications are essentially related to the devascularization of the distal part of the donor common duct when it is too long or extensively debrided. Depending on its intensity, distal ischemia leads to either necrosis or stenosis of the duct's end. Necrosis occurs a few days after the transplantation when immunosuppression is at its highest level, thus increasing the risk of death. It results in a bile leak with bile peritonitis or with biloma formation in the subhepatic area. Biloma can remain undetected for weeks or months before it becomes infected with anaerobic bacteria or fungus. Fibrosis of the distal part of the duct leads to stenosis and obstruction of the biliary tract. It is revealed by cholangitis episodes, cholestatic syndrome or, ultimately, intrahepatic biliary tract dilatation.

Other exceptional causes of biliary obstruction, e.g. unknown lithiasis of the recipient duct or stenosis of the sphincter of Oddi, have been reported. Exceptionally, bilirubinate gallstone causes obstruction, in patients with hemolysis or when liver transplantation has been performed across ABO blood group barriers. Particular attention must be paid to the extrinsic compression of the donor's cystic duct by a mucocele. This mucocele appears when both the proximal and distal ends of the cystic duct have been occluded [5]. Such a phenomenon occurs when the cystic duct enters the common duct at the site of anastomosis, but it can be avoided by leaving the proximal end of the cystic duct opened.

Finally, complications related to the presence of a stent in the lumen still require special attention because of their high occurrence rate, especially with T-tube drainage in the choledoco-choledocostomy reconstruction. These complications include leaks at the exit site, dislodgement, biliary obstruction and infection [2]. In our experience, biliary reconstruction complications represent 88 % of all biliary complications. They are reported in Table I.

Table I. Biliary reconstruction complications following liver transplantation in our series of 286 cases.

Biliary anastomosis	Biliary reconstruction complications			
	Leaks*	Stenosis*	Drain related	
			Leaks	Obstructions
CC *n* = *212*	8 (22)	11 (30)	8 (22)	6 (16)
CJ** *n* = *74*	3 (8)	1 (3)	0	0
Total *n* = *286*	11 (30)	12 (32)	8 (22)	6 (16)

CC = Choledocho-choledochostomy ; CJ = Choledocho-jejunostomy.
( ) = % of total number (n = 37) of biliary reconstruction complications.
* At the anastomosis site ; ** 21 were pediatric cases.

Ischemic biliary complications are related to the loss of arterial supply to the graft biliary tract.

Thrombosis of the hepatic artery represents the leading cause of ischemic biliary complications. This is due to the fact that the hepatic artery is the sole supplier of blood to the extra- and intra-hepatic ducts. Thrombosis is generally caused by a technical error such as an inadequate anastomosis, intimal dissection or arterial angulation. Ischemic biliary complications are characterized by bile duct strictures which affect only the graft biliary tree, and which are separated by intrahepatic biliary leakages ; these leakages are due to the total destruction of the biliary wall and closely resemble dilatations on cholangiograms. These lesions can be multiple or single, and generally occur within months following the transplantation.

Since Doppler ultrasound is available and can be performed routinely, it appears that thrombosis of the hepatic artery does not necessarily lead to ischemic biliary complications. This phenomenon can be explained by the fact that a microarterialization of the graft, growing from the surrounding tissues, i.e. the jejunal limb of the choledocho-jejunal anastomosis, may develop with time. The more intense the neovascularization, the less thrombosis of the hepatic artery will induce biliary repercussions. Thus, while early thrombosis of the hepatic artery leads to serious ischemic biliary complications associated with hepatic failure, late thrombosis of the hepatic artery may be either totally asymptomatic (20 % of the cases) or less symptomatic (isolated intrahepatic stricture). The preservation of neovascularization is important when conservative therapy has been chosen upon.

Five cases of ischemic type biliary complications occurred in our 286 OLTs (12 % of 42 biliary complications). In the first two cases, thrombosis of the hepatic artery occurred immediately after transplantation, and caused an anastomotic leak with hepatic failure. The two patients died of multiple organ failure. In the next two cases, hepatic artery thrombosed at the anastomosis site and ischemic type biliary complication occurred 6 and 8 months after transplantation, respectively. One patient had strictures localized on the extra-hepatic duct and was treated conservatively with a hepatico-jejunostomy. The other patient developed extensive destruction of the biliary tree with multiple parenchymal abscesses and required an emergency retransplant. The fifth case showed a thrombosis of the right branch of the hepatic artery and subsequent destruction of the right biliary tree. A second OLT was carried out, but the patient died of multiple organ failure.

Recently, new type of biliary complications has been identified following liver transplant [6]. They have also been called « ischemic type biliary complications » because they exhibit the cholangiographic features described earlier, but they occur in the absence of thrombosis of hepatic artery, chronic rejection or ABO blood group incompatibility. They have been shown to be associated with the extended preservation time of the graft (> 13 h in the UW solution). But like other teams [7], we have never been confronted with this type of biliary complication, even with preservation times of up to 25 hours.

Infections of the biliary tree are not primitive, and viral (CMV) or fungal cholangitis similar to those complicating acquired immune deficiency syndrome, have never been reported. Bacterial cholangitis frequently accompanies ischemic or technical complications and may be due to a cholangiography through an infected T tube.

Immunological biliary complications have been reported in two different situations. The first occurs following liver transplants across ABO blood group barriers [8], where a progressive and diffuse destruction of the biliary tree, similar to that seen in sclerosing cholangitis, takes place within 4 to 6 months after the operation while the hepatic artery is patent. It is likely that this phenomenon is immunologically mediated, even if the exact underlying mechanisms have yet to be found. The second, a total destruction of biliary ducts, is often associated with chronic rejection (only 3 cases, 1 %, in our experience). It has been suggested that two mechanisms could be responsible for this « vanishing bile duct syndrome » : direct immunologic damage, probably antibody mediated, and ischemia, due to the obliteration of micro and macro arterial vasculature of the ducts, secondary to a fibrointimal hyperplasia [7].

Diagnostic strategies

Prompt recognition can markedly decrease the morbidity and mortality of biliary complications. However, this is quite difficult since clinical or biological signs specifically related to biliary complications are lacking. Most of the time, clinical profiles associate liver dysfunction with clinical deterioration (fever, ileus, ascites) that might also be related to rejection, preservation injury, generalized sepsis, cyclosporine toxicity or any other metabolic complication that may occur following liver transplantation. For this reason, an algorithmic use of diagnostic modalities is required.

When a T tube or an internal stent is still present, a cholangiogram should be performed immediately. A Doppler ultrasound must be used to confirm hepatic artery patency. If the biliary tree cannot be opacified promptly and easily, ultrasound should be performed. It can easily detect intra or subhepatic fluid collection that can be punctured percutaneously in order to confirm the diagnosis, and opacify the collection. As a first step, the collection can be drained percutaneously. Exploration of the hepatic artery, using Doppler ultrasound or angiogram, is mandatory.

Ultrasonography is not particularly accurate in the early detection of biliary dilatation, and unless clinical or histological findings clearly indicate any other causes of liver dysfunction, it is necessary to visualize the biliary tree. Invasive opacification by endoscopic retrograde cholangiopancreatography (ERCP) or percutaneous transhepatic cholangiography (in case of choledoco-choledocostomy or choledoco-jejunostomy, respectively) is required in order to exclude or confirm biliary complication.

Therapeutic strategies

Once the diagnosis of the biliary tract complication is established, specific therapy should be immediately implemented.

Therapeutic options for biliary reconstruction complications management may be non-operative if end-to-end choledoco-choledocostomy was chosen for the bile duct reconstruction. A biloma may require the simple reopening of a T tube or percutaneous drainage, associated with ERCP sphincterotomy [10]. A stenosis of the duct-to-duct anastomosis can be dilated by ERCP or percutaneously [11]. However, if complications occur early after transplantation, or if there is an important bile duct defect, or if the first choice for biliary reconstruction was a choledoco-jejunostomy, external maneuvers can be dangerous and an operative approach to reconstruct the anastomosis higher in the hepatic hilum is preferable. Extensive destructions of the extrahepatic biliary system has been successfully treated with cholangio-jejunostomy [12].

Ischemic biliary complications are more difficult to manage. Conservative treatment (intrahepatic biloma drainage, percutaneous dilatations and stenting, hemihepatectomy or hepatico-jejunostomy) is indicated when liver function is good and infection eradicated with proper antibiotherapy. In other cases, retransplantation is usually necessary.

More interesting would be the development of biliary reconstruction techniques that could decrease the incidence of biliary complications following transplantation. Reduction of graft preservation time, good assessment of duct vascularization and optimal choice of the best recipient site for artery anastomosis represent a first step in this direction. These can only improve with surgical experience. Since a large number of biliary reconstruction complications were related to the use of a T tube, the role of choledocho-choledochostomy anastomosis without a T tube has been evaluated in a retrospective study [2] that showed a lower complication rate when the T tube was omitted. We are now prospectively evaluating this technique and a preliminary analysis of our data suggests that even if drain-related complications have disappeared, they have been replaced by an increased number of post-operative stenosis, leading to reoperation.

*

* *

In conclusion, biliary tract complications following liver transplantation are still common (14.5 % of our transplant cases) but most of them are benign if a prompt diagnosis is made. Long-term results of non-operative treatments have yet to be assessed. Complications that jeopardize liver function are unfrequent ; they are related to liver ischemia and generally justify retransplantation.

References

1. Klein SA, Savader S, Burdick JF, Fair J, Mitchell M, Colombani P, *et al.* Reduction of morbidity and mortality from biliary complications after liver transplantation. Hepatology 1991 ; 14 : 818-23.
2. Rough DA, Emond JC, Thistlethaite JR, Mayes JT, Broelsh CE. Choledochocholedochostomy without a T tube or internal stent in transplantation of the liver. Surg Gynecol Obstet 1990 ; 170 : 239-44.
3. Lerut J, Gordon RD, Iwatzsuki S, Esquivel CO, Todo S, Tzakis A, *et al.* Biliary tract complications in human orthotopic liver transplantation. Transplantation 1987 ; 43 : 47-51.
4. Krom RAF, Kingma LM, Haagsma EB, Wesenhagen H, Slooff MJH, Gips CH. Choledochocholedochostomy, a relatively safe procedure in orthotopic liver transplantation. Surgery 1985 ; 97 : 552-6.
5. Koneru B, Zajko AB, Sher L, Marsh JW, Tzakis A, Iwatsuki S, *et al.* Obstructing mucocele of the cystic duct after transplantation of the liver. Surg Gynecol Obstet 1989 ; 168 : 394-6.
6. Sanchez-Urdazpal L, Gores GJ, Ward EM, Maus TP, Wahlstrom HE, Moore SB, *et al.* Ischemic-type biliary complications after orthotopic liver transplantation. Hepatology 1992 ; 16 : 49-53.
7. Adam R, Bismuth H, Diamond T, Ducot B, Morino M, Astracioglu I, *et al.* Effect of extended cold ischemia with UW solution on graft function after liver transplantation. Lancet 1992 ; 340 : 1313-6.
8. Gugenheim J, Samuel D, Reynes M, Bismuth H. Liver transplantation across ABO blood group barriers. Lancet 1990 ; 336 : 519-23.
9. Oguma S, Belle S, Starzl TE. A histometric analysis of chronically rejected human liver allografts : insights into the mechanism of bile duct loss ; direct immunologic and ischemic. Hepatology 1989 ; 9 : 204-9.
10. Ward EM, Wiesner RH, Hughes RW, Krom RAF. Persistent bile leak after liver transplantation : biloma drainage and endoscopic retrograde cholangiopancreatographic sphincterotomy. Radiology 1991 ; 179 : 719-20.
11. Zajko AB, Campbell WL, Bron KM, Lecky JW. Iwatsuki S, Shaw BW, *et al.* Cholangiography and interventional biliary radiology in adult liver transplantation. Am J Roentgenol 1985 ; 144 : 127-33.
12. Langnas AN, Stratta RJ, Wood RP, Ozaki CF, Bynon JS, Shaw BW. The role of intrahepatic cholangiojejunostomy in liver transplant recipients after extensive destruction of the extrahepatic biliary system. Surgery 1992 ; 112 : 712-8.

Progress in Hepatology 93. J.P. Miguet and D. Dhumeaux, eds.
John Libbey Eurotext, Paris © 1993, pp. 135-143

15

New perspectives in liver transplantation

H. BISMUTH, L. CHICHE

Hepatobiliary Surgery and Liver Transplant Research Unit, South Paris University, Faculty of Medicine, 94804 Villejuif, France.

Since the first human liver transplantation was performed in 1963 [1], the procedure has been progressively developed and refined and is now routinely performed in most of the developed countries throughout the world. Initial results were variable and generally disappointing but several major developments, including improvements in organ procurement and preservation, refinement of the technical aspects and advances in anaesthesia and intensive care, resulted in a gradual improvement in results in the 1970s. One of the most major breakthroughs has been the introduction of the immunosuppressive agent cyclosporine [2]. Following the dramatic improvement in long-term survival using this and a decision by the Consensus Development Conference of the National Institutes of Health in the United States of America (June 1983), that liver transplantation had become a service and was no longer simply an experimental procedure, there has been a marked annual increase in the number of transplantations performed not only in the USA, but also in Europe and in the rest of the developed world [3-5].

Indications for liver transplantation cover an astonishing range of diseases

Liver transplantation may be considered for any patient with progressive or acute liver disease which is likely to terminate fatally with other standard treatment options. Transplantation has now been performed for virtually all liver diseases but the main indications are cirrhosis, paediatric diseases and cancers. The indications may be classified according to the type of the disease, for example, parenchymal, cholestatic or neoplastic (Table I). In recent years, there has been a slight change in indications for liver transplantation, the most notable trends being an increase in the proportion of post-hepatitic cirrhosis in the cirrhotic group, with a corresponding decrease in the proportion of primary biliary cirrhosis, an increasing proportion of transplantations for fulminant hepatitis, an increasing proportion of re-transplantations, a slight increase in alcoholic cirrhosis as an indication and a decreasing proportion of transplantations for hepatocellular carcinoma and other primary hepatic cancers [4, 5]. The age range of patients in which transplantation may be indicated has also changed, with the procedure now being regularly performed in small infants and patients over 60 years [4, 5].

Table I. Indications for liver transplantation.

Parenchymal disease

- Post-hepatitic cirrhosis
- Alcoholic cirrhosis
- Fulminant hepatitis
- Budd-Chiari syndrome
- Congenital hepatic fibrosis
- Cystic fibrosis
- Neonatal hepatitis
- Hepatic trauma

Cholestatic disease

- Biliary atresia
- Primary biliary cirrhosis
- Secondary biliary cirrhosis
- Sclerosing cholangitis
- Familial cholestasis

Inborn errors of metabolism

Tumours

- Benign
- Primary malignant
- Metastatic : endocrine tumours
  : non-endocrine tumours

Recent developments

Following the introduction of cyclosporine and the acceptance of liver transplantation as a clinical service, the development of the technique has progressed so rapidly that it may now be performed almost as a routine procedure. One of the most significant advances has been the development of a new solution (University of Wisconsin (UW) solution) for preservation of the liver during the cold ischaemia period (the period between clampage of the blood supply in the donor and revascularization in the recipient). This, unlike the previously used Euro-Collins solution, permits preservation and storage of the liver for up to 20 hours [6]. This has transformed the practice of liver transplantation, with the recipient operation now being performed as a semi-elective procedure in some centres [7]. The prolonged cold ischaemia allowed by the use of UW solution also has several other major advantages such as more appropriate matching between donor and recipient, procurement and transport of grafts from distant locations (even trans-atlantic) and the ability to prepare a second patient for transplantation should the findings at laparotomy in the first (for example, extrahepatic malignancy) indicate that transplantation is not feasable. In addition, newer techniques such as graft size reduction and graft « splitting » for transplantation of 2 patients may be performed in a more leisurely fashion [8, 9].

The use of reduced size grafts, first discussed by one of us (HB) for heterotopic transplantations, is a technique employed when the graft is too large for the fossa into which it is to be placed. The most obvious example is the transplantation of a child or small infant with a liver from an adult [8]. Precise knowledge of the functional anatomy of the liver, with the individual blood supply and biliary drainage of each liver segment [10], together with new techniques such as ultrasonic dissection of the liver, has allowed this to be performed with relative safety and good results [8, 11].

This concept has been taken one stage further with the development of liver « splits ». This was first performed by Pichlmayr [12] and Bismuth [13] in 1988 and since then has been performed in several other centres [9]. The main indication for the technique at present is the transplantation of two patients, one child and one adult, with one needing an urgent transplantation. There are, however, a significant number of complications associated with procedure and results are not yet as good as for transplantation of whole or reduced size livers but with further advances and experience these should improve [9]. The possibility to have two distinct teams associated to use the two parts of the liver makes the procedure less heavy.

Following the development of reduced size and split liver transplantation, the next development involved the use of modern techniques in liver surgery to remove a part of the liver from a living donor for transplantation into a recipient related to the donor (living-related donation). The first successful living-related liver transplant was performed in Australia, followed by a larger series in the USA [14, 15] and Japan [16]. The main indication for living-related liver donation is the presence of fulminant hepatitis or severe end-stage chronic liver failure where a cadaveric donor is not available. Another situation in which this technique has been used is to allow liver transplantation in countries such as Japan where the law at present prevents cadaveric organ donation. The ethical issues surrounding living-related donation are important in terms of the risk to the donor but for equivalent operations (left lobectomy) in non-jaundiced, non-cirrhotic patients the morbidity rate is low and the mortality may be considered as nul in our center as in other specialized centers.

Current problems

One of the major problems in the use of liver transplantation for the treatment of end-stage liver disease at present is the availability of cadaveric donors. Donor availability has become a major problem in recent years with the marked expansion in the number of liver transplantations being performed and expansion of the range of indications, while at the same time there has been a relative decrease in the number of potential donors, with improved road safety and compulsory wearing of seat belts. While newer developments such as split liver grafting and living-related donation may ameliorate the problem to some extent, it is unlikely to match the current demand for donors. Presently, in France, approximately 71 % of patients with end-stage liver disease have to wait 0 to 6 months for a suitable liver graft while 25 % have to wait 7 to 12 months and 4 % have to wait 13 to 24 months [17]. It seems certain that the number of patients and the waiting period will increase considerably in the next 5 to 10 years. Unfortunately, for end-stage liver disease there is no temporising form of treatment analogous to renal dialysis.

Another major problem at present in terms of overall survival following liver transplantation is the recurrence of native disease in the grafted liver [3]. This is particularly true for transplantation for malignant liver disease. The other disease which frequently recurs in the transplanted liver is hepatitis B although it has been recently shown that the incidence of this can be reduced by long-term passive anti-HBV immunoprophylaxis [18].

Rejection remains one of the major problems in liver transplantation. While the prohibitively poor survival secondary to rejection has been overcome by the introduction of cyclosporine and combination immunosuppression regimens [19], acute and chronic rejections are still a major cause of graft failure and graft loss. The most commonly used combination of drugs to prevent rejection is cyclosporine and steroids, supplemented in some centres by azathioprine [19]. For acute rejection episodes bolus injections of steroids or the monoclonal antibody OKT3 may be used. A newly introduced immunosupressive agent, FK506, has shown promising results in laboratory studies and in one center (Pittsburgh), and is currently undergoing extensive evaluation in clinical studies [3].

Sepsis with subsequent multiple organ failure is a significant cause of morbidity and mortality following liver transplantation. This is related principally to immunosuppression especially in patients debilitated by a long standing disease but also to the magnitude of the procedure with the necessity for extensive invasive monitoring.

Future techniques and developments

The future for liver transplantation in Europe and in the world seems to be related to the advancement and implementation of recently developed techniques such as split liver grafting and at a less extent living-related donation. Advances in immunosuppressive therapy and in the treatment of sepsis and multiple organ failure, possibly with newly introduced endotoxin antibodies [20], may improve results. Auxiliary heterotopic liver transplantation (transplantation of the liver in the abdomen with the patient native liver still *in situ* [21], particularly of isolated hepatic sectors or segments, may also be further developed. The problem of the limited donor pool may be partly overcome by split liver grafting and living-related donation. Increasing the age for acceptance of a patient for donation may also help address this problem [3]. However, with the increasing indications for liver transplantations, particularly post-hepatitic cirrhosis, alcoholic cirrhosis, and transplantation of more patients at the extremes of the age spectrum, the demand for donors will also increase. Most developed countries now have liver transplantation programmes sufficient to meet their needs and these will, no doubt, continue to increase in size. For the countries which presently do not have the capacity to provide this service (for example, small countries and some of the developing countries), refinements and advances in the procedure and the postoperative and general care of these patients may make it a viable proposition. In countries where cadaveric organ donation is not permitted (e.g. Japan) there will probably be a significant expansion in living-related liver transplantation within the next few years. As total substitutions of the livers by a prothetic organ is presently not only unrealisable but also unconceivable, xenografting is the ultimate goal, presently in the field of intensive research.

In the last few years, there has been a resurgence of interest in xenotransplantation, which appeared to be a future solution to the shortage of organs and to other problems such as the recurrence of virus B on grafts. As a matter of fact, xenotransplantation is a potentially important source of organs which could be easily available. The donor could be chosen and prepared, the transplantation electively organized. Nevertheless xenotransplantation still rises a large amount of unsolved problems : choice of the donor species, control of the xenogenic rejection, knowledge and control of the infectious risks, metabolic functionality, ethical approval.

In fact, those problems are more or less crucial, depending on the type of xenograft performed, i.e. on the donor for a human recipient. Yet in the sixties, two situations had been individualized : the discordant xenotransplantation (performed in widely related species) and the concordant xenotransplantation (performed in closely related species) [22, 23]. In the first case, there are preformed natural antibodies against the donor and the rejection is hyperacute, that is strong and immediate. In the second case, there is a certain immunological compatibility and the absence of preformed natural antibodies against the donor : the rejection is strong but delayed [24].

Two models were and are still intensively studied in man :

Non-human-primate to man xenotransplantation

Chimpanzees and baboons were used in clinical xenotransplantations in humans in the sixties [25-29], the eighties (Bailey) [30], and recently by Starzl [31]. Immunological, anatomical and physiological conditions are probably optimal concerning chimpanzee-to-man transplantation, and previous renal xenotransplantation from chimpanzee to man in the sixties with unsophisticated immunosuppression had shown it. Baboons are smaller animals, and immunologically more distant from human, but they are more easily available. The recent cases of Starzl and coll. of a baboon to human liver transplantation [31] proved their ability to control xenogeneic rejection and the capacity of a baboon liver to replace functionally the human organ. Nevertheless, several problems remain unsolved : the real availability of such animals as far as xenotransplantation programs are concerned (chimpanzees are protected and cannot be used, baboons are easily bred in captivity but gestation time is long and only adults are usable), the infectious problems (primates, even bred in captivity, may harbor simian viruses potentially dangerous for man), the ethical issues (moral acceptability of breeding and killing those animals so close to us, reaction of animal liberationists...) [32].

The model pig to man

It has several advantages : the availability of numerous and controlled animals is greater, organs from pigs are anatomically concordant to man's, size between recipient and donor can be easily matched, the existing use of pigs for human use makes the acceptance of breeding centers for xenotransplantation easier. Nevertheless, one of the major problems is the immunological incompatibility in this model, and our incapacity to control definitely hyperacute rejection. Another problem in case of liver xenotransplantation is the functionality of a xenogeneic organ.

In fact, for the moment, xenotransplantation seems to be acceptable if, in a particular case, no other alternative source of organ is available. For example, in Starzl recent case which was quite well accepted in the scientific and public opinion, the justification of the liver xenotransplantation was the viral hepatitis infection of the recipient which could be transmitted to any human graft but not to baboons hepatocytes. So in the future, because of the real need of organs to save human lifes, xenotransplantation can be justified but with some restrictions : selection of the indications of such transplantations in respect to animal life is mandatory, progress in the different immunological and infectious problems of xenotransplantation is awaited, and ethical approval is needed in public and scientific opinion.

General conclusions

Since the first human liver transplantation was performed almost 30 years ago, the procedure has advanced rapidly and has become a widely used method for the treatment of end-stage liver disease in the developed world. It has provided the opportunity of prolonged life (some patients now surviving for more than 20 years) to patients who would otherwise certainly have died. Developments in the technique have led not only to many breakthroughs in liver surgery and transplantation, but also to advances in other areas such as immunology, anaesthesia, metabolism, intensive care, and the management of multiple organ failure. The quality of life which most people enjoy following transplantation is excellent with 85 % of patients able to return to the community and to perform their jobs well [3]. Long-term survival results depend on the indication for transplantation and are best for children with metabolic diseases and biliary atresia, but even for adults the 3-year survival following elective transplantation for cirrhosis is approximately 75 %. These figures continue to improve each year [4, 5, 33].

References

1. Starzl TE, Marchioro TL, Von Kaulla KN, *et al.* Homotransplantation of the liver in humans. Surg Gynecol Obstet 1963 ; 117 : 659.
2. Calne RY, Rolles K, White DJG, *et al.* Cyclosporine A initially as the only immunosuppressant in 34 recipients of cadaveric organs : 32 kidneys, 2 pancreases and 2 livers. Lancet 1979 ; 2 : 1033-6.
3. Starzl TE, Demetris AJ, Van Theil D. Liver transplantation. N Engl J Med 1989 ; 321 : 1092-9.
4. Bismuth H, Castaing D, Ericson BG, Otte JB, Rolles K, Ringe B, Sloof M. Hepatic transplantation in Europe. First report of the European Liver Transplant Registry. Lancet 1987 ; 2 : 674-6.
5. European Liver Transplant Registry. December 1991 updating. Hôpital Paul Brousse, 94800 Villejuif, France.
6. Kalayoglu M, Sollinger HW, Stratta RJ. D'Alessandro AM, Hoffmann RM, Pirsch JD, Belzer FO. Extended preservation of the liver for clinical transplantation. Lancet 1988 ; 1 : 617-9.
7. Todo S, Nery J, Yanga K, Podesta L, Gordon RD, Statzl TE. Extended preservation of human liver grafts with UW solution. JAMA 1989 ; 261 : 711-4.
8. Bismuth H, Houssin D. Reduced-sized orthotopic liver graft in hepatic transplantation in children. Surgery 1984 ; 95 : 367-70.
9. Edmond JC, Whitington PF, Thistlethwaite JR, Cherqui D, Alonso EA, Woodle IS, Vogelbach P, Busse-Henry SM, Zuker AR, Broelsch CE. Transplantation of two patients with one liver. Analysis of a preliminary experience with « split-liver » grafting. Ann Surg 1990 ; 212 : 14-22.
10. Couinaud C. Le foie : études anatomiques et chirurgicales. Paris : Masson, 1957.
11. Bismuth H. Surgical anatomy and anatomical surgery of the liver. World J Surg 1982 ; 6 : 3-12.
12. Pichlmayr R, Ringe B, Gubernatis G, Hauss J, Bunzendahl H. Transplantation of one donor liver to two recipients (splitting transplantation). A new method for further deve-

lopment of segmental liver transplantation. Langenbecks Arch Chir 1988 ; 373 : 127-30.
13. Bismuth H, Morino M, Castaing D, Gillon MC, Descorps Declere A, Saliba F, Samuel D. Emergency orthotopic liver transplantation in two patients using one liver. Br J Surg 1989 ; 76 : 722-4.
14. Strong RW, Lynch SV, Ong TH, Matsunami H, Koido Y, Balderson GA. Successful liver transplantation from a living donor to her son. N Engl J Med 1990 ; 322 : 1505-7.
15. Broelsch CE, Edmond JC, Whitington PF, Thistlethwaite JR, Bucker AL, Lichtor JL. Applications of reduced-size transplants as split grafts, auxiliary orthotopic grafts and living-related segmental transplants. Ann Surg 1990 ; 212 : 368-75.
16. Yamaoka Y, Ozawa K, Tanaka A. New devices for harvesting hepatic graft from the living donor. Transplantation 1991 ; 52 : 157-60.
17. France Transplant. Rapport annuel. Bulletin n° 8. April 1991.
18. Samuel D, Bismuth A, Mathieu D, Arulnaden JL, Reynes M, Benhamou JP, Bréchot C, Bismuth H. Passive immunoprophylaxis after liver transplantation in HBsAg-positive patients. Lancet 1991 ; 337 : 813-5.
19. Gugenheim J, Samuel D, Saliba F, Castaing D, Bismuth H. Use of cyclosporine in combination with low dose steroids and azathioprine in liver transplantation. Transplant Proc 1988 ; 20 : 3.
20. Ziegler EJ, Fisher CJ, Sprung CL, *et al.* Treatment of Gram-negative bacteremia and septic shock with HA-lA human monoclonal antibody against endotoxin. A randomized double blind placebo controlled trial. N Engl J Med 1991 ; 324 : 429-36.
21. Houssin D, Franco D, Berthelot P, Bismuth H. Heterotopic liver transplantation in end-stage HBsAg-positive cirrhosis. Lancet 1980 ; 1 : 990-3.
22. Perper RJ, Najarian JS. Experimental renal heterotransplantation : I. In widely divergent species. Transplantation 1966 ; 4 : 377-88.
23. Perper RJ, Najarian JS. Experimental renal heterotransplantation : II. Closely related species. Transplantation 1966 ; 4 : 700-12.
24. Hammer C, Suckfull M, Saumweber D. Evolutionary and immunological aspects of xenotransplantation. Transplant Proc 1992 ; 24 : 2397-400.
25. Bach FH. Xenotransplantation : a view to the future. Transplant Proc 1993 ; 25: 1-9.
26. Reemtmsa K, McCracken BH, Schlegel JV, *et al.* Renal heterotransplantation in man. Ann Surg 1964 ; 160 : 384-408.
27. Starzl TE, Marchioro TL. Renal heterotransplantation from baboon to man. Transplantation 1964 ; 2 : 752-76.
28. Wegman R, Léger L, Monsallier F, *et al.* Histo-chimie d'une greffe hétérotopique d'un foie de babouin sur une patiente atteinte d'hépatite fulminante. Presse Med 1970 ; 78 : 403-8.
29. Barnard CN, Wolpowitz A, Lossman JG, *et al.* Heterotopic cardiac transplantation with a xenograft for assistance of the left heart in cardiogenic shock after cardiopulmonary bypass. South Afr Med J 1977 ; 52 : 1035-8.
30. Bailey LL, Nelhsen-Cannarella SL, Conception W, *et al.* Baboon-to-human cardiac xenotransplantation in a neonate. JAMA 1985, 254 ; 23 : 3321.
31. Starzl TE, Fung J, Tzakis A, *et al.* Baboon-to-man liver transplantation. Lancet 1993 ; 341 : 65.
32. Singer P, Frey RG. Animal rights and animal research. In : Beauchamp TL, Pinkard L, eds. Ethics and public policy. Englewood cliffs : Prentice-Hall, 1983 : 387.
33. Bismuth H, Farges O, Samuel D, Castaing D. Past, present and future in liver transplantation immunosuppression. Transplant Proc 1992 ; 24 : 85-7.

Achevé d'imprimer par Corlet, Imprimeur, S.A.
14110 Condé-sur-Noireau (France) - N° d'Imprimeur : 9655 - Dépôt légal : août 1993
Imprimé en C.E.E.